*INFANTS
AT
RISK*

Summary Publications in the Johnson & Johnson Baby Products Company Pediatric Round-Table Series:

Maternal Attachment and Mothering Disorders: A Round Table

Edited by Marshall H. Klaus, M.D.,
   Treville Leger, and
   Mary Anne Trause, Ph.D.

Social Responsiveness of Infants

Edited by Evelyn B. Thoman, Ph.D.,
   and Sharland Trotter

Learning Through Play

By Paul Chance, Ph.D.

The Communication Game

Edited by Abigail Peterson Reilly, Ph.D.

Infants at Risk: Assessment and Intervention

Edited by Catherine Caldwell Brown

INFANTS AT RISK

Assessment and Intervention

An Update for Health-Care Professionals and Parents

Edited by
Catherine Caldwell Brown

*Summary of a Pediatric Round Table,
"New Approaches to Developmental
Screening of Infants,"
Chaired by T. Berry Brazelton, M.D.
Chief, Child Development Unit
The Children's Hospital Medical Center
Boston, Massachusetts*

with

*Barry M. Lester, Ph.D.
Director, Developmental Research
Child Development Unit
The Children's Hospital Medical Center
Boston, Massachusetts*

Introduction by
T. Berry Brazelton, M.D.

Sponsored by
Johnson & Johnson
BABY PRODUCTS COMPANY

Copyright © 1981 by Johnson & Johnson Baby Products Company

All rights reserved. No part of this book may be reproduced in any form, by photostat, microform, retrieval system, or any means now known or later devised, without prior written permission of the copyright holder.

Library of Congress Cataloging in Publication Data
Main entry under title:

Infants at risk.

   (Johnson & Johnson Baby Products Company pediatric round table series; 5)
   "Summary of a pediatric round table chaired by T. Berry Brazelton . . . with Barry M. Lester."
   1. Child development — Testing — Congresses. 2. Infant psychology — Congresses. 3. Child development deviations — Congresses. I. Brown, Catherine Caldwell. II. Johnson & Johnson Baby Products Company. III. Pediatric Round Table on New Approaches to Developmental Screening of Infants (1980: Palm Beach, Fla.) IV. Series. [DNLM: 1. Child development — Congresses. 2. Child development disorders — Congresses. WS 105 I42 1980]
RJ51.D48I53   618.92   81-11755

ISBN 0-931562-06-6   AACR2

Printed in the United States of America

For all those who help infants at risk grow up

Contents

List of Participants	ix
Preface	xiii
Introduction T. Berry Brazelton, M.D.	xv
Editor's Introduction	xxi
PART I — NEW WAYS IN ASSESSMENT	xxiii
Optimality: A New Assessment Concept Heinz F. R. Prechtl, M.D.	1
Neurological Examination of the Neonate for Silent Abnormalities S. Saint-Anne Dargassies, M.D.	5
Gestational Age, Birth Weight, and the High-Risk Infant Lula O. Lubchenco, M.D.	12
The Continuity of Change in Neonatal Behavior Barry M. Lester, Ph.D.	18
Assessing Infant Individuality Heidelise Als, Ph.D.	24
Toward a Model of Early Infant Development Frances Degen Horowitz, Ph.D.	31
Neurophysiological Assessment of the Neonate Frank H. Duffy, M.D.	40
Early Screening for Developmental Delays and Potential School Problems William K. Frankenburg, M.D.	48
Predicting Developmental Outcome: Resumé and Redirection Robert B. McCall, Ph.D.	57

PART II — EARLY INTERVENTION: SOME STRATEGIES   71

Intervention Programs for Infants with Cerebral Palsy: A Clinician's View
    Lawrence T. Taft, M.D.   73

Early Intervention for Preterm Infants
    Arthur H. Parmelee, Jr., M.D.   82

An Ecological Approach to Parent-Child Relations
    Kathryn E. Barnard, R.N., Ph.D.   89

Intervention Strategies Using Temperament Data
    William B. Carey, M.D.   96

The Intimate Relationship of Health, Development, and Behavior in the Young Child
    Martin Bax, M.D.   106

A Sensory-Motor Enrichment Program
    Eric Denhoff, M.D.   113

Participants

HEIDELISE ALS, Ph.D.
Assistant Professor of Pediatrics
  (Psychology)
Harvard Medical School and
Director of Clinical Research
Child Development Unit
The Children's Hospital Medical Center
300 Longwood Avenue
Boston, MA 02115

KATHRYN E. BARNARD, R.N., Ph.D.
Professor of Nursing
School of Nursing
University of Washington
Seattle, WA 98195

MARTIN C. O. BAX, M.D.
Thomas Coram Research Unit
41 Brunswick Square
London WC1
ENGLAND

T. BERRY BRAZELTON, M.D.
Associate Professor of Pediatrics
Harvard Medical School and
Chief, Child Development Unit
The Children's Hospital Medical Center
300 Longwood Avenue
Boston, MA 02115

MS. CATHERINE CALDWELL BROWN
Science Writer
105 Somerville Road
Ridgewood, NJ 07450

WILLIAM B. CAREY, M.D.
319 W. Front Street
Media, PA 19063

ERIC DENHOFF, M.D.
Clinical Professor of Pediatrics
Brown University Medical Program
293 Governor Street
Providence, RI 02906

MR. JAMES T. DETTRE
Director, Marketing Services
Johnson & Johnson
  Baby Products Company
220 Centennial Avenue
Piscataway, NJ 08854

FRANK H. DUFFY, M.D.
Associate Professor of Neurology
Harvard Medical School and
Director of Developmental Neurophysiology
Department of Neurology
The Children's Hospital Medical Center
300 Longwood Avenue
Boston, MA 02115

WILLIAM K. FRANKENBURG, M.D.
Professor of Pediatrics and Preventive
  Medicine
Director, John F. Kennedy
  Child Development Center
University of Colorado
Health Sciences Center
4200 East Ninth Avenue
Denver, CO 80262

FRANCES DEGEN HOROWITZ, Ph.D.
Professor of Human Development, Psychology
Department of Human Development
University of Kansas
Lawrence, KS 66045

BARRY M. LESTER, Ph.D.
Assistant Professor of Pediatrics
  (Psychology)
Harvard Medical School and
Director of Developmental Research
Child Development Unit
The Children's Hospital Medical Center
300 Longwood Avenue
Boston, MA 02115

LULA O. LUBCHENCO, M.D.
Professor of Pediatrics - Emerita
University of Colorado
Health Sciences Center
4200 East Ninth Avenue
Denver, CO 80262

ROBERT B. McCALL, Ph.D.
Senior Scientist and Science Writer
Boys Town Center
Boys Town, NE 68010

ARTHUR H. PARMELEE, JR., M.D.
Professor of Pediatrics
Department of Pediatrics
University of California
Center for the Health Sciences
Los Angeles, CA 90024

HEINZ F. R. PRECHTL, M.D.
Professor and Director
Department of Developmental Neurology
University Hospital
Oostersingel 59
9713 EZ Groningen
THE NETHERLANDS

MR. ROBERT B. ROCK, JR., M.A., M.P.A.
Director, Professional Relations
Johnson & Johnson
 Baby Products Company
220 Centennial Avenue
Piscataway, NJ 08854

DOCTEUR S. SAINT-ANNE DARGASSIES
Maitre de Recherches
Directeur Adjoint
du Centre de Recherches Neonatales
de l'Association Claude-Bernard
Laureat de l'Academie Nationale de
 Medecine
123, boulevard de Port-Royal
75674 Paris Cedex 14
FRANCE

STEVEN SAWCHUK, M.D.
Director, Medical Services
Johnson & Johnson
 Baby Products Company
220 Centennial Avenue
Piscataway, NJ 08854

MR. ROBERT C. STITES
President
Johnson & Johnson
 Baby Products Company
220 Centennial Avenue
Piscataway, NJ 08854

LAWRENCE T. TAFT, M.D.
Professor and Chairman
Department of Pediatrics
Rutgers Medical School, CMDNJ
P.O. Box 101
Piscataway, NJ 08854

Preface

In our previous Round Table on "Language Behavior In Infancy and Early Childhood," we were fascinated by the manner in which language development served as an indicator of the presence or absence of a variety of childhood disabilities. We were even more intrigued by the prospects of using language development in developmental screening as a diagnostic tool for predicting the child at risk. This led us, quite naturally, into the subject of the fifth in the series of Johnson & Johnson Baby Products Company Pediatric Round Tables, "New Approaches to Developmental Screening of Infants," chaired by T. Berry Brazelton, M.D.

In fostering this series, the company continues to provide support for scholarly reviews of the state of the art which bring to child health-care professionals and interested parents new concept information and insights at the innovative edge of child development. *INFANTS AT RISK: Assessment and Intervention,* written and edited by Catherine Caldwell Brown, is the summary publication based on the material presented at this fifth Round Table. It has been reviewed and edited by the chairperson and by the other participating professionals.

In *INFANTS AT RISK: Assessment and Intervention,* Catherine Caldwell Brown has concentrated attention on the diverse, yet related, contributions of 15 of the world's authorities in this fascinating area of child development. The first part of the book considers new approaches to assessment techniques; the second part reviews strategies for their application to early intervention. In addition to effective communication between the professional in clinical practice and the parents of the child at risk, the participants in this Round Table highlight the all-pervasive influence of socioeconomic status (SES) and the child's home environment. They also consider the impact of SES on variables relating to the infant and the infant/parent relationship and, in turn, to child development. In the consideration of such concepts, together with exploration of specific intervention techniques, the explanation of related assessment instruments, and the review of positive professional attitudes toward intervention programs, the publication of this summary volume seeks — through transfer of its insights and information — to help child health-care professionals, together with parents, to expand the future for infants at risk.

Robert B. Rock, Jr., M.A., M.P.A.
Director of Professional Relations

Introduction
by T. Berry Brazelton, M.D.

The Round Table summarized in this book gathered together some leading researchers and practitioners in the field of infant assessment and intervention. The many disciplines represented — pediatrics, neurology, neurophysiology, nursing, developmental psychology — are a testimony to the breadth of this field.

The questions we tried to confront are also broad. How urgent is the need for early identification of infants at risk for developmental failure? Do the dangers of labeling outweigh the advantages of intervention? What opportunities for recovery of function do early identification and early intervention provide?

At present, it seems, practicing physicians tend to postpone the referral of damaged infants to intervention programs. The United Cerebral Palsy Foundation, which has been instituting early intervention programs in various parts of the country, reports a disturbing statistic: if one waits for a pediatrician to refer a cerebrally damaged infant, the mean age at referral is 14 months; if parents self-refer, infants arrive by 4 months of age. Obviously, such a statistic has many inherent problems and biases, but it does make a point.

Physicians may postpone a diagnosis of central nervous system (CNS) damage or of developmental lag "to protect parents," or they may be defending themselves against the recognition of CNS damage because it is something they can do little about. Yet in my experience parents' suffering is not increased by early identification of an infant's problems. On the contrary, early identification offers support to parents who already sense they are in trouble. All caring parents inevitably experience a grief reaction, which probably deepens if they can't find confirmation or support from the physicians and nurses to whom they bring their child. But parents are marvelously successful at turning grieving around. When their perceptions are taken seriously and they receive support from a professional, they can take the energy that had been expended on self-recrimination and feelings of helplessness and put it to work in the service of the baby.

Parents of at-risk babies certainly profit by early identification and intervention, but what about the infants? What are the possibilities for recovery or functional plasticity in an infant with a known CNS insult? Ian St. James-Roberts (1979) describes several pathways for apparent plasticity or recovery of function in the developing CNS.

1. *Vicarious functioning.* A separate or functionally dormant brain area takes over the function, resulting in the resumption of normal behavior. This model, described by Munk in 1881, does not rely on environmental intervention, but it does demand an immature brain.

2. *Equipotentiality.* Proposed by Lashley in 1938, this model assumes considerable redundancy in the CNS, and mass action of many units rather than specified centers. It allows for takeover by substitution of equipotential centers. The extent of recovery by this process would depend on the site and extent of lesions. Luria (1970) talks of inhibited pathways that are redundant and can be called upon. A nurturing environment might foster the organization necessary to call up these pathways' function.

3. *Substitution.* Behavioral substitution can sometimes achieve the same goals as the function that has been lost. Meyer (1974) reviews ways that interference in lesion areas can be compensated for by using functions of intact areas. An environment that permits regression and allows time for recovery would certainly increase the likelihood of effective substitution.

4. *Regrowth and supersensitivity* of neurons after injury. Regenerative sprouting of damaged axons involving the original neuron may help compensate for an injury. The idea of supersensitive neurotransmitters that' "leak" into the damaged area and activate post-lesion

pathways with restoration of normal action is intriguing but still controversial. If the leakage is too great, overcompensation and hypersensitivity with resultant ineffectual function can also occur. Perhaps overcompensation occurs in an overstimulating environment. This possibility fits well with the notion that "appropriate stimulation" is a source of organization toward recovery whereas "inappropriate stimulation" is an overload that interferes with recovery.

5. *Diaschisis.* This model rests on the idea that trauma interferes with neural systems by causing general disruption of the CNS (surrounding irritation or hematoma, changes in cerebrospinal fluid and composition, edema, vascular supply changes, and so on). As the disruptive reactions subside, the neural systems of an immature CNS may have a better chance of recuperation and even of invasion and takeover by surrounding plastic systems. Functional bewilderment or generalization of reduced function may also be present, and from this the baby will recover. In this model, the environment's capacity to provide stimuli that will help the infant organize his or her behavior (rather than overwhelming the child) will be critical.

Sameroff and Chandler (1975) suggest a sixth model: a succession of stages in which progress is followed by reorganization. This *"jagged progress" model* includes successive spurts and reorganizations not only of the baby's internal function but of the environment's efforts to achieve "normalcy" or "optimality." It rejects a critical period hypothesis as too rigid and replaces it with a more dynamic one in which there is reorganization, regression, and re-energizing before each spurt of improvement. This model appeals to me; it reflects my experience.

An infant's own capacity for recovery at an organic and functional level can be fostered through appropriate external experience. In the same way, an environment that overwhelms a child or provides inappropriate stimulation can retard his or her progress. If we believe these assertions are true, how do we help the environment provide energy toward recovery?

To achieve a nurturing environment for the child, we must be sensitive to the needs of the parents as they face the violation of their hopes and expectations that a damaged infant represents. I have never been as struck with the importance of this aspect of intervention as when I visited the Meeting Street School, a multidisciplinary intervention project for CNS-damaged infants in Providence, Rhode Island. The emphasis there is on the parents' involvement with the child as a total person. The treatment of damaged systems is considered less important than the functional recovery of intact systems.

When we entered the school to observe, I noticed a severely impaired 3-year-old with continuous athetotic movements of all extremities lying on a mattress across the room. She saw me standing with her teacher and with the director, Dr. Eric Denhoff, and called out across the room, "Hi, come here." I waved politely and said hello but did not obey. Very firmly, she repeated, "I said, come *here!*" Her imperious tone had power, and this time I went. The child's confidence in her ability to command showed me that her self-image had been fostered and preserved in spite of her CNS impairment. When a professional staff backs up parents in a way that leads them to preserve a child's self-image, this fosters the child's inner motivations for progress toward recovery — no matter what the defects or how severe.

Whether a child is normal, at risk, or obviously impaired, an assessment does more than provide a momentary glimpse of his or her functioning. The child's performance on a test, examined within the conceptual framework of organizational stages suggested by Sameroff and Chandler, also offers insight into the child's past and future. By giving credence to the baby's style, temperament, and way of coping with the demands of the test situation, we can learn a great deal about the infant.

In our Unit at Boston Children's Hospital, our best use of assessment is as intervention. Each assessment in which parents participate does automatically become an intervention. By participating *with* parents in the identification of the child's strengths and weaknesses, and by sharing with parents the information we gain, we can help them distinguish stimuli that are appropriate and can be utilized from stimuli likely to overwhelm the child. We can share with parents our working understanding of the child's internal organization and response systems and try to channel their energy and understanding of the child toward optimization of function. We can certainly enhance the power of a nurturing environment to provide opportunities for plasticity. Perhaps most important of all, we can reinforce their self-image as parents so that they in turn can nurture their child's.

The papers that follow reflect the challenge of this potential both for "recovery" and for compensation for deficits. The parents' treatment of the child is probably the most important element in the child's image of himself or herself as a competent person — despite any organic deficit.

Editor's Introduction

The views expressed at our Round Table were at least as diverse as the professional fields represented by the participants. Science is only beginning to become acquainted with the human infant, and the gaps in our knowledge about this mysterious creature leave plenty of room for differences of opinion. In addition, it became increasingly clear as the conference proceeded that many of the issues surrounding infant assessment and intervention are social as well as scientific, with implications for public policy. No wonder the participants spoke with many voices!

Consider two findings. First, as reported in the paper by Frank Duffy, roughly half of all infants born very early and below the expected weight for their gestational ages will have learning difficulties during childhood. Second, as reported in the paper by William Frankenburg, about half the infants born into poverty circumstances will also have learning problems after entering school.

This provocative pair of statistics raises many questions that were discussed during our conference. Among them:

1. Are the outlooks for populations facing biological (or medical) risk and social risk really so similar? How do they differ?

2. At present, there is no reliable way to tell which half of either population will do well and which less well. What progress is being made in developing more informative assessment instruments?

3. Are similar intervention strategies for the two risk populations desirable? Feasible?

4. Considering the many unknowns, is it appropriate to treat risk groups at all? Perhaps one should wait for definite current symptoms. What is the difference between a "risk factor" and a "symptom"?

5. On a clinical basis, how can the practitioner best respond to the needs of individuals from either of these risk groups (or any other)?

In editing the round-table proceedings, my primary purpose was to maintain the integrity and coherence of each participant's perspective on such questions. For that reason, the discussion that follows each paper is presented as a dialogue, with the speaker's name preceding his or her remarks. If readers find themselves interrupting the conversation, so much the better — the heuristic purposes of our round table will be served.

Secondarily, I tried to retain the information that seemed most likely to enhance the clinical efforts of practitioners. Issues of infant assessment and intervention, like so many issues confronting those in clinical practice, are still largely matters of judgment. Readers must draw their own conclusions about infants at risk — who they are and what to do about it. I hope this book will help with this fascinating but difficult process.

Catherine Caldwell Brown

PART ONE
NEW WAYS IN ASSESSMENT

Optimality:
A New Assessment Concept
by Heinz F. R. Prechtl, M.D.

The best way to predict which infants will probably develop cerebral palsy, mental retardation, or other problems involving the central nervous system might seem to be by looking at early risk factors — very low birth weight, for example, or severe oxygen deprivation (hypoxia) at birth. However, this method of prediction does not work well. The great majority of newborns who are at risk, for whatever reason, develop normally. The fact that it is so difficult to predict faulty development from any neonatal risk sign, and therefore so difficult to avert it through early intervention, is a problem that came up repeatedly at our conference.

Heinz Prechtl has found an ingenious solution: instead of assessing risk, assess what he calls "optimality." Infants who are in very good shape at birth almost always develop well. Thus, Prechtl says, the optimality scale has good predictive power. The scale assesses prenatal factors, including the mother's health, as well as characteristics of the newborn.

Prechtl lives in the Netherlands and was unable to attend the round table. His paper, which is summarized below, was read by Barry Lester.

The dream still lives that a way can be found to identify newborn infants who will later suffer physical or mental handicaps caused by damage to the nervous system. The usual approach to this prediction problem attempts to relate risk factors, in the form of pre- and perinatal complications, to later developmental abnormalities. However, the predictive power of these risk factors is poor.

An example will illustrate some of the difficulties. An Apgar score of 0-3 at five minutes, which is generally accepted as a serious sign of postnatal depression, occurs some 22 times more often in infants who will be severely handicapped as children than in others. However, the same Nelson and Broman study that yielded this finding also showed that 96.5% of all infants with 0-3 Apgar scores develop normally. Thus, the prediction of severe later impairment is correct for only about 3.5% of cases.

In clinical practice, knowledge of obstetrical complications is indispensable for identifying the etiology of certain conditions of the newborn infant, and the clinician must continue to use diagnostic categories of complications in daily routine and research. A cause-effect relationship between pre- and perinatal complications, however, should not be assumed without sufficient evidence.

Early abnormal neurological signs (symptoms and syndromes) are stable from day to day but very rarely persist in their original form over a long period of time. Most either disappear permanently or change their nature and appearance. Others give way to a prolonged symptomless period followed by different symptoms. This variability in early neurological signs, which may be related to age-specific properties of the developing nervous system, further complicates the prediction problem.

THE PREDICTIVE POWER OF OPTIMALITY. For purposes of prediction, the optimality approach to assessment gives better results than traditional obstetric complications scales. Though it may seem trivial when low-risk neonates are found to be neurologically normal or even optimal, the prognostic value of such findings is not at all trivial. A normal neonatal neurological finding has a higher predictive value for later normality than does any abnormal sign for later abnormality. If the obstetrical history includes risk factors but the neonatal neurological findings are normal, the likelihood of later normality is still very high.

The criteria for optimality have been carefully and strictly defined. A comprehensive list covers social, maternal, fetal, and infant data, including such items as maternal age, parity, maternal blood pressure, condition of the placenta, fetal position, fetal heart rate, spontaneous delivery, birth weight, onset of breathing after birth, gestational age, and course of postnatal adaptation. The various lists in use include 40 to 70 of such well-defined items.

For each item that meets the predetermined criteria, a point is added to the infant's score. For items not in agreement with optimality criteria, points are lost. Since only one point is given per item, a significant decrease in optimality is only possible if several items are not optimal. It has been found empirically that reduced optimality on certain "important" items is usually accompanied by reduced optimality on other factors. Therefore, the scale is self-weighting.

Although the optimality scale has important advantages over traditional complications scales, it also has limitations. Its greatest drawback is that the gain in quantification may be accompanied by a loss of qualitative information concerning existing risk factors. This loss can easily be overcome by using both types of scale: the optimality scale for prediction and the complications scale for diagnosis and etiology. When both types of scale are used, a consistent result is that only in infants showing reduced optimality does the complication under consideration (maternal hypertension, for example) have adverse effects on the nervous system. Thus, the optimality score captures the complexity of obstetrical conditions.

A quite different limitation derives from the difficulties people may have thinking in terms of optimality. The approach is very unfamiliar to medical people, who are trained to search for abnormalities and pathology. The optimality concept is not merely a reversal of the complications concept but is essentially different from it. On many items, the optimum is more narrowly defined than the normal. Consequently, conditions of reduced optimality may fall within the limits of normality, or they may indicate severe pathology.

It would be a serious mistake to conclude from my

stress on the predictive power of optimality that a diagnosis of early brain dysfunction is unimportant. Even if a later neurological impairment is found in only a small percentage of cases showing early dysfunction, there may be deviant development in other complex patterns of behavior, such as social bonding. Further, neurological conditions in the young infant must be appreciated in their own right, not evaluated solely in the light of long-term effects. Even transient dysfunctions of the nervous system should not be considered trivial or clinically insignificant.

In conclusion, it should be pointed out that the aim of neurological assessment differs from that of behavioral assessment. The two methods are complementary. They measure different aspects of the child and therefore cannot replace each other. This distinction must be fully appreciated in order to make rational intervention and treatment possible.

Carey: Could someone clarify the difference between Prechtl's optimality score and a complications score? Evidently they aren't just opposites.
Parmelee: As an example, take maternal age. You can't say that having a very young mother is pathological, but you can say that it is more normal, or optimal, to have a mother whose age is within a certain range.
Lubchenco: I have to agree with Prechtl that we physicians are geared to pathology more than to normality, and that we ought to try looking the other way.
Brazelton: From a clinician's standpoint, an optimality score has the advantage of emphasizing the strengths rather than the weaknesses of the infant at risk. It is all too easy for parents to concentrate on the negatives. Perhaps scoring the baby for positives would help the parents develop positive expectations, which might then become a self-fulfilling prophecy.
Parmelee: Still, in judging the predictive power of abnormal signs we sometimes forget that when we

find a problem like respiratory distress in a neonate, we treat it immediately. To the extent that we're successful in our therapy, we confound our indices.

Frankenburg: I wonder what the group would think about looking not only at child variables, which Prechtl emphasizes, but at family variables and society variables. In trying to predict child development, it seems to me that all three areas, and particularly the rate of change in each, would be key. For instance, if a child is biologically impaired and not progressing, that is a bad sign. If the child's family is not adapting to the problem, that's doubly bad. And if society doesn't value children who are unwell, then the child faces a triple risk.

Brazelton: As we look for alternatives to an "either/or" model of neurological damage, it seems to me we do need an interactional model that includes family and social factors. Perhaps we can work toward that as our discussion proceeds.

*Examination of the Neonate for Gestational Age and Silent Neurological Abnormalities**

by S. Saint-Anne Dargassies, M.D.

The new science of neonatology is abandoning an old word: premature. *The word is becoming obsolete because it is imprecise. It makes no distinction between an infant born early (now called preterm) and an infant born light (now called small-for-gestational-age or small-for-date). The distinction is a good one, for the outlooks of the two groups are not identical, but it does create a problem. How is the pediatrician to establish an infant's gestational age at birth without relying on the*

---

*Adapted from The normal and abnormal neurological examination of the neonate: silent neurological abnormalities. In R. Korobkin and C. Guilleminault (Eds.), *Advances in Perinatal Neurology* Vol. I. New York: SP Medical and Scientific Books, 1979.

outdated criterion of weight or last maternal menstruation?

In the paper that follows, S. Saint-Anne Dargassies describes a quick, five-step neurological assessment that she has developed for evaluating gestational age. She also discusses infant neurological development and the need to examine infants for silent, or hidden, neurological abnormalities. Although she could not attend our round table, she sent two of her training films, one showing her examination of preterm infants for gestational age and one detailing silent neurological signs in full-term infants.

A newborn infant is assumed to be neurologically normal if weight, appearance, breathing, crying, and sucking are normal for the presumed gestational age, and if the primary reflexes (Moro, rooting, walking) are present. However, because of the presumed normality, a cursory examination may fail to identify silent or latent prenatal lesions that place later development at risk. Even in the face of apparent normality, then, a systematic and methodical search should be made for silent pathology.

The purpose of a neurological examination of the neonate is to recognize any symptomatological impairment. Unfortunately, one cannot always ascertain the location or extent of a lesion, or even its pathology, by clinical pediatric examination. Thus, the goal becomes one of recognizing dysfunction in the central nervous system (CNS), whether transient or permanent. The dysfunction may be minimal at first, yet indicate a deep-seated disorder which may manifest itself belatedly or appear as evidence of an acute insult.

EXAMINATION FOR MATURATION. Figure 1 shows the contrast between an infant's responses at 28 and 41 weeks gestational age. Table 1 explains how to assess fetal age clinically, in a simplified examination based on five signs. The newborn can remain in a supine position throughout this simplified examination; if it seems desirable, the examination can be conducted

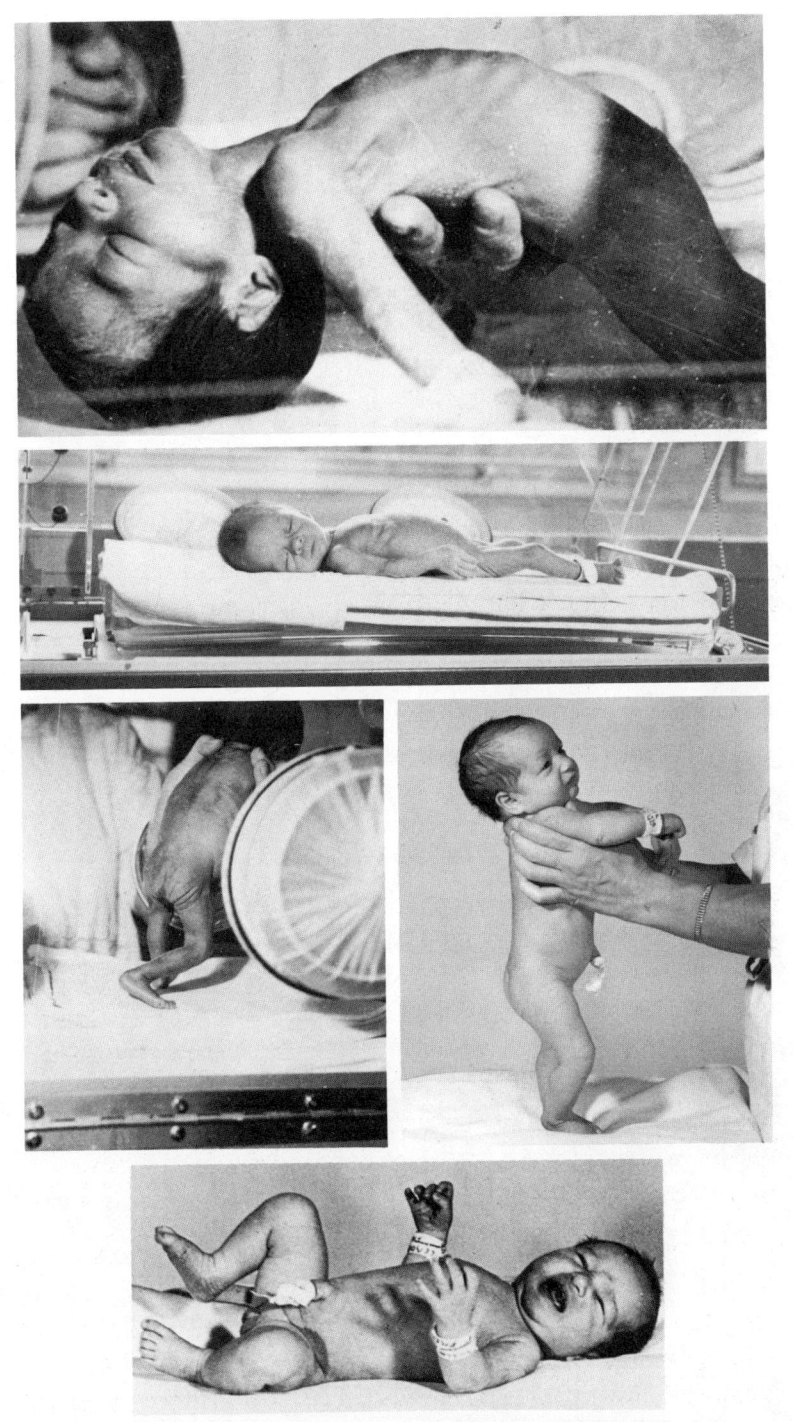

Figure 1. Contrast between infant responses at 28 and 41 weeks gestational age.

TABLE 1.

	28 weeks	30 weeks	32 weeks	35 weeks	37 weeks	41 weeks
Resting posture	Total extension of 4 limbs. Head rests on side of face.	Extension of 4 limbs. Chin touches acromion.	Extension of upper limbs. Slight flexion of popliteal joint. Chin inside acromion.	Legs flexed, thighs abducted, extension of arms. "Frog" posture.	Flexion of 4 limbs. Chin well ahead of acromion.	Equal and powerful flexion of 4 limbs. Chin near sternum.
Crossed adductor reflex	No reaction or repetitive defense gesture with long reaction time.	Defense and retraction movement more localized, of lesser amplitude. Inhibited by cry.	Extension with very wide abduction.	Abduction more limited during passive extension. Fanning of toes.	Linked flexion, then extension. Extension is prolonged and dominates.	3rd phase: adduction, free foot comes up and then moves close to stimulated foot, sometimes over it.
Angle of foot	35°	35°	40°	30°	15° (except in former prematures)	0° (except in former prematures)
Difference in tone between upper and lower extremities	When lifted then released, the 4 limbs fall limply with no rebound.	Passive fall of the legs with slight rebound.	Disappearance of limp, passive fall of legs.	Excellent recoil of legs; excessive hypotonia of arms with limp, passive fall.	Recoil in arms possible but inhibited by slow, prolonged downward extension.	Brisk, sudden recoil of 4 limbs. Equal resistance in arms and legs.
Cardinal reflexes (rooting)	Lateral response must be aided by holding head. Only lips participate.	Holding head no longer indispensable. Head extension added to lateral response.	Lateral response immediate, brisk, repetitive. Head extension distinct. Outline of flexion.	3 phases: lateral, repetitive, extension of head. Participation of lips, tongue and head.	Improvement of 4th phase, flexion of head, but it remains limited.	4 phases are equally perfect. Head movements easy and equal amplitude in all 4 directions.

while the infant is lying in the incubator. The clinician records the response observed for each of the five investigations by checking the square in the lower right-hand corner of the space. These marks should normally be evenly distributed down the column corresponding to one fetal age. When the five responses are distributed in two adjacent columns, this indicates that the infant belongs to the intermediate age.

The evaluation of maturity by determination of gestational age is important for three reasons. First, the neurological picture changes with age, and the same response can be normal at one stage and pathological at another. Poor head control, for instance, may be considered normal in a preterm infant but abnormal in a small-for-gestational-age term infant.

Second, gestational age must be determined so that we can correctly evaluate later development. Third, a strict check for gestational age will enable us to detect small-for-date infants, who are at risk for neonatal disorders and later abnormalities but who are so often confused with preterm infants.

EXAMINATION FOR SILENT NEUROLOGICAL ABNORMALITIES. The major signs of neurodevelopmental disorder include: (1) poor or absent vigilance (the quality of alertness that allows an infant to be receptive and to react appropriately to tactile, auditory, or visual stimuli); (2) abnormal motility — an absence of spontaneous activity, an excess of movement, or bursts of abnormal movements; (3) pathological ocular signs, such as fixed or deviated eyeballs; (4) abnormal tone of the neck or trunk muscles — for example, poor head control when the child is moved from supine to sitting position and back again; (5) a cry that is abnormal in tone; and (6) straightening reactions.

Pathological signs must be grouped into clusters to permit the diagnosis of syndromes. Minor symptoms, when multiplied and grouped, can constitute a signal for close surveillance. Such clusters may also lead to the belated diagnosis of a condition that was latent in earliest life, or that was incorrectly attributed to another cause.

Deviant evolution may exist from the start or develop later, or there may be a gradual aggravation of silent cerebral malformations or hereditary, metabolic, or genetic diseases with no clearly defined dysmorphism. Dysmorphic features are often absent in the neonate only to become obvious slowly, with maturation. Initial symptomatic impairment is the early signal of a need for complementary investigations (such as laboratory tests) and for continuing careful observation. The period of uncertainty can span at least the first two years of life, for time is sometimes needed to define the syndromes that throw light on the past and future of the infant and lead finally to a true diagnosis.

CONCLUSION. In neonates, serious abnormalities are sometimes undetectable and may remain so for some time. Obvious perinatal impairments may conceal or mask the deeper underlying cause of a subsequent disastrous evolution.

Despite a normal clinical appearance, minor neurological signs that are grouped into clusters may reveal a silent syndrome that is decisive for the quality of later development. The infant must be examined carefully and repeatedly over a period of time. One must note associated clinical signs and then seek appropriate complementary laboratory or radiological studies.

Prenatal factors, though silent, exist at birth and can sometimes be detected neurologically. Systematic and thorough semiological investigation of all newborns would advance our knowledge of prenatal factors that from an early date determine the quality of an infant's future.

Editor's note. The discussion below followed a film, made by Saint-Anne, showing her periodic examinations of premature infants from 26 to 41 weeks gestational age. This film and others by Saint-Anne can be obtained by writing to F.A.C.S.E.A., 972 Fifth Avenue, New York, NY 10021.

Brazelton: These are obviously very powerful films,

beautifully done. They're also brave, in that Saint-Anne is trying to correlate alertness and neuromuscular maturity with gestational age. If you use the grids that she has devised (Table 1), you can place a newborn according to reflex behavior, muscle tone, and so on, and reach a conclusion about maturational age that does not depend on birth weight.

Parmelee: Saint-Anne's techniques and recommendations are based on her clinical observations rather than on empirical studies, you know. From about 1950 on, she's looked at premies every day of her life — she probably has more experience with them than anyone at this table. It may be a particularly French idea that looking at individual cases for 30 years tells you much more than looking at groups for a year and quantifying the information.

Lester: She does have an underlying theory, though, a plan involving primary reaction patterns and global organizations in the baby. In addition, her textbook (Saint-Anne Dargassies 1977) describes the computerized analysis of some of her findings.

Lubchenco: What do you think about putting a tiny premie like the one in the film through such a taxing examination? In most nurseries today, that baby would have an IV and be in an isolette, not really accessible for this kind of examination.

Brazelton: The film we saw was for teaching purposes only. Saint-Anne would never recommend that such an examination be performed routinely. Routine clinical evaluation, she says, must be based only on the five-step procedure shown in Table 1. You'll notice that the procedure requires the examiner to manipulate the baby's limbs but not to lift the child out of a supine position. One reason Saint-Anne chose the rooting reflex for use in this short exam is that it is easy to elicit while the infant is lying down.

Parmelee: I'm not an expert on newborn examinations,

but I have watched Saint-Anne a few times and she is marvelous at controlling the baby. Every time the infant gets the least bit upset, she calms it down immediately. She also does partial exams when they're indicated, which is less tiring for the infant. It's hard to pin her down on just why she chose to do a particular part of the exam on a particular child at a particular time, though.

Brazelton: Certainly we all must be very, very careful in working with preterms and small-for-dates. I still get scared when I think of an incident I was responsible for some years ago. I was demonstrating a premature baby's attentional behavior to the mother. The baby was wonderful, following my face and turning to my voice, and I got so excited that I overlooked the signs of exhaustion that someone like Saint-Anne is in tune with all the time. All of a sudden, the baby stopped breathing and had to be incubated again. This baby had given plenty of warning signals, I realized later. I think these signs should be taught to mothers, by the way, and certainly to all the professional people who deal with these tiny babies.

Gestational Age, Birth Weight, and the High-Risk Infant

by Lula O. Lubchenco, M.D.

The newborn's "vital statistics" — gestational age, weight, length, and head circumference — are the subject of Lula O. Lubchenco's paper. These statistics, particularly when considered in relation to each other, convey much information. For example, a small-for-gestational-age infant with a relatively large head circumference has a better prognosis than an infant of the same gestational age and weight with a small head circumference. The latter infant is more likely than the former to have a congenital infection or anomaly.

In discussing neonatal diseases, Lubchenco points out that a newborn who is ill or under stress may seem lethargic and withdrawn. Before clear symptoms develop, the infant may fail to eat well, respond weakly to stimuli, and become jittery if disturbed. Relatively unresponsive behavior is also characteristic of preterm infants who are not ill. As later papers point out, such behavior can create problems as parents try to establish a relationship with their baby.

It is becoming routine in this country to evaluate infants for gestational age at birth. A formal scoring system like that of Dubowitz may be used, though from a practical standpoint an abbreviated form is usually satisfactory. An infant's weight, length, and head circumference at birth are easily obtained. Examined together, these parameters provide significant information on the likelihood of mortality, morbidity, and even specific morbidity.

Neonatal mortality is lowest in infants born at term with birth weights somewhat above the mean. The highest mortality rate occurs in those with the lowest birth weights and shortest gestational ages. Mortality rates have been declining in recent years, following improvements in intrapartum and neonatal care.

Long-term morbidity in very high-risk infants has also declined. Apparently the same effort and supports that make it possible for the infant to survive also protect the brain and give the infant a better chance for normal growth and development. The relationship between birth weight and long-term outlook is far less clear, however, than the relationship between birth weight and mortality. A new variable, medical management or intervention in the form of aggressive intrapartum and neonatal care, helps account for this.

BIRTH WEIGHT. Specific morbidities can be anticipated from the percentile standing of a newborn infant on the intrauterine growth curve. Large-for-gestational-age infants now have a good prognosis. Their mortality

NEWBORN CLASSIFICATION AND NEONATAL MORTALITY RISK
BY BIRTH WEIGHT AND GESTATIONAL AGE

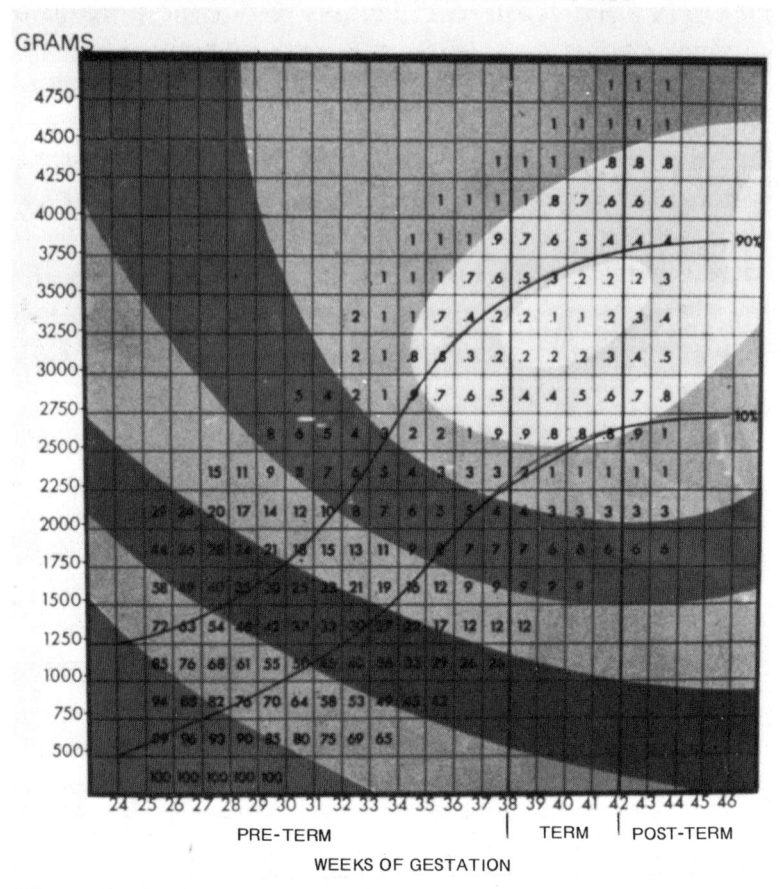

Figure 2. Newborn Classification and Neonatal Mortality Risk.

is near zero. Common morbidities include those associated with a diabetic mother, especially when she gives birth before term. Genetically large infants delivered at term may also be at risk, and post-term normal infants must be watched for birth trauma.

Many more conditions are associated with intrauterine growth retardation than are associated with increased fetal growth. Partly for this reason, the small-for-gestational-age infant presents a diagnostic problem. Some of the questions that arise can be answered easily; others are more difficult.

A review of the prenatal history will show whether

the mother was toxemic or hypertensive. Prolonged, severe toxemia and hypertension result in small infants. Various other maternal diseases and conditions also reduce fetal growth, but not necessarily below the tenth percentile. These include maternal undernutrition, smoking, alcohol or drug ingestion, low socioeconomic status, living at high altitudes, and being very young or very old from an obstetric viewpoint.

HEAD CIRCUMFERENCE. When evaluating potential problems in the small-for-gestational-age infant, the other body measurements are helpful. The small-for-gestational-age infant with a relatively large head compared to weight or length is likely to have problems of hypoglycemia and polycythemia but has a good prognostic outlook. The small-for-gestational-age infant with a small head circumference compared to length is more likely to have congenital anomalies or infections and a less good prognosis. All small-for-gestational-age infants are subject to intrapartum stress, so that obstetric management is crucial.

Another method for evaluating morbidity at various birth weights and gestational ages is to map the incidence of specific conditions by birth weight and gestational age. Congenital heart disease, for example, occurs at a much higher rate in small-for-gestational-age infants than in others. Hypoglycemia, though it occurs most often in small-for-gestational-age infants and next most often in preterm infants, is also found in full-term infants of average weight. Such infants tend to have low Apgar scores at birth or a wasted appearance.

Similar symptoms occur in hypoglycemia, hyperviscosity, sepsis, pneumonia, and many other neonatal diseases. It is as if newborns have a limited ability to respond to stress or illness. Their first response, which may appear as lethargy, closed eyes, and poor feeding, is to "withdraw" or "turn off" stimuli. These infants become jittery if disturbed. When they can no longer "turn off" the stress, overt symptoms appear.

The assessment techniques used with newborns at our hospital include nurses' observations, the Brazelton

Neonatal Behavioral Assessment Scale (1973), and routine laboratory screening for glucose and polycythemia. The Brazelton scale identifies sick infants, but reaching a specific diagnosis usually requires laboratory documentation.

Treatment for hypoglycemia is easy once the condition is identified, and outcome is improved over previous years. Treatment of hyperviscosity is not so easy, though partial plasma exchange to decrease blood viscosity appears to be helpful in reducing the severity of symptoms in the first two weeks.

In summary, many high-risk infants can be identified by birth weight/gestational age criteria. Neonatal symptoms are usually present in sick or stressed infants when examined in the manner prescribed by Brazelton. However, the symptoms are general and differ from the "classic" ones seen in older infants and children, making them hard to interpret. Increased recognition of illness and improved diagnostic techniques will likely improve the long-term outlook for this population.

Brazelton: What about identifying small-for-gestational-age infants before birth? Would that help, and can it be done?

Lubchenco: Our obstetricians can pick up about half of the small-for-dates, using ultrasound and other measures, but whether and how to act on the information is another question. At this time they don't deliver early just because the baby is small, though they may if tests of fetal well-being show the infant is in trouble.

McCall: A small-for-date infant is at greater risk than a preterm infant even if both weigh the same, is that right?

Lubchenco: Generally, yes. But judging from our experience, small-for-date infants don't necessarily have the poor outcome that some people, particularly Fitzhardinge, have found. I think it's significant that Fitzhardinge's population was a transport population. The infants were born in community hospitals, which probably had few facilities for fetal monitoring and stabilization. At our hospital, small-for-dates are watched very carefully during labor and have a good outlook. In fact, when we looked at infants with birth weights under 1500 grams (3.3 pounds), we found a slightly higher percentage of normal infants in the small-for-date group than in the preterm group.

Bax: Has the rate of small babies in the United States been declining? It seems to me that better nutrition, better obstetrics, and better care for newborns should mean fewer small babies. But in the United Kingdom, in spite of our marvelous health service, we still get about 7% small babies. The Scandinavians do better, with 5%.

Lubchenco: According to the Colorado State Health Department, the percentage of infants in the state who weigh 2500 grams or less at birth seems to be holding steady at 8 or 9%.

Brazelton: Here's something I've wondered about, partly because of my experiences in Guatemala. Both chronic prenatal stress like maternal malnutrition and acute stress or trauma can result in a small baby. But are there other differences in their effects?

Lubchenco: That's an interesting idea. We don't see much malnutrition at our hospital, but preliminary data suggest that babies with malnourished mothers may have smaller heads and a less good prognosis than, say, babies from mothers with toxemia or hypertension, where the head seems to grow relatively better than length and weight.

Brazelton: In Guatemala we saw two syndromes. One appeared in term infants whose weight was right but who looked obviously immature. These babies always ended up short. I worried a lot about these babies because they seemed to have been chronically stressed. The other appeared in infants born to women whose placentas gave out at the end of pregnancy. They were acutely small-for-date looking and acting, but somehow less worrisome than the first group.

Bax: I recall a study in which the researchers used ultrasound to measure intrauterine head growth, and they found that infants whose heads seemed to stop growing at 33 weeks were much worse off than those whose heads stopped growing in the last two weeks.

Lubchenco: A disproportionately small head circumference is always a bad sign, a clue that you need to look for infection or anomaly in the baby.

The Continuity of Change in Neonatal Behavior
by Barry M. Lester, Ph.D.

The Neonatal Behavioral Assessment Scale (NBAS), developed by T. Berry Brazelton and his colleagues over a period of 20 years, was the first major behavioral scale for use with newborns. Though it assesses reflexes, it is not primarily a neurological exam. It engages the newborn in interaction with the examiner and points up especially the infant's efforts to control his or her own environment.

A criticism sometimes made of the NBAS is that infants tend not to receive the same scores when tested repeatedly over a period of time. In the first of three papers on new work with the Brazelton scale, Barry Lester argues that infants' scores vary because change is characteristic of the newborn period. Using computerized statistical techniques, Lester and his coworkers have identified several patterns of change that seem to typify the behavior of neonates (as reflected in their NBAS scores). Particularly in preterm infants, these patterns can be related to performance on the Bayley Scales of Infant Development in later infancy.

The neonatal period is characterized by rapid changes in behavioral development as the infant recovers from the stress of labor and delivery and adapts to the postnatal caregiving environment. The instability of neonatal behavior has frustrated researchers and clinicians who are interested in assessment. "How can we measure something if it keeps changing?" they ask. "How can we predict later development from newborn behavior if newborn behavior itself is unstable?"

Most assessment models are based on the assumption that what we want to measure is stable. What is not stable is regarded as noise in the system, or error. We assume, for example, that a 7-year-old child's IQ should be virtually the same from day to day. But for neonates, change rather than stability may be the rule. Jerome Kagan has even argued that change is the dominant characteristic of infancy, and that there may be few if any connections between the structures of successive stages. Kagan uses the analogy of embryonic cells that vanish after they complete their function and, like scaffolding for a building, are no longer needed.

NEONATAL BEHAVIORAL ASSESSMENT SCALE. The instrument we have used in studying neonatal change is the Brazelton Neonatal Behavioral Assessment Scale (NBAS). The Brazelton scale, which is itself based on a dynamic model of infant behavior, assesses 20 reflexes and includes 26 behavioral items. The reflex exam is used to manipulate the infant's state (asleep, drowsy, awake, crying) and to interact with the baby rather than as part of a comprehensive neurological evaluation. If more than three deviant reflexes are noted (excluding those that are not expected to be well developed at birth), a separate neurological exam is in order.

The 26 behavioral items cover response decrement; orientation to social and nonsocial stimuli; motor maturity and tone; variation in state, color, and activity level; self-quieting abilities; and social behavior such as smiling and cuddling. The behavioral scale is conceptualized as an interaction between the baby and the examiner, and it gives special attention to newborn behaviors that are salient in interactions with parents.

Playing the role of caregiver, the examiner takes the baby through a range of states and situations that call for adaptive strategies, always trying to elicit the infant's best (not average) performance. A successful examination requires sensitivity to the baby's cues and an ability to manipulate the baby's behavior. For example, the infant should be brought through the repertoire of state changes as smoothly as possible.

During the first months of life, behavior as assessed by the Brazelton scale changes dramatically. If day-to-day stability as measured by traditional psychometric methods is the criterion, then as a testing instrument the NBAS falls short. However, if change and not stability is the hallmark of the neonatal period (and perhaps of infancy in general), then an instrument that reflects change, as does the NBAS, may have great value.

Brazelton himself has stated repeatedly that high stability on the NBAS should not be expected. It is the baby's pattern of change over repeated assessments, he says, that should predict developmental outcome.

PATTERNS OF CHANGE. For the past few years we have been developing a statistical method and computer-scoring routine for describing and quantifying patterns of individual differences over repeated examinations on the Brazelton scale. The study of these fluctuations is not part of the conventional statistical bag of tricks, and our method is complex. Briefly, factor analysis and other statistical procedures are used to generate curves for each infant that represent the individual infant's pattern of change across several exams. The single items of the Brazelton scale are summarized into clusters for each exam: habituation, orientation, motor performance, range of state, regulation of state, autonomic regulation, and reflexes. A curve is computed for each cluster that describes how the infant changed on that cluster over the series of exams. Each curve is then computer-scored along parameters that describe the shape of the curve, how much change was shown, and whether the infant improved or not and by how much over the repeated exams. These parameters can then be used to compare individuals and groups.

It appears from our work to date that these curves (sometimes called "recovery curves") do represent patterns of individual differences in the organization of neonatal behavior and that these patterns differ between term and preterm infants. Further, data from a longitudinal study suggest that the patterns may be related to developmental outcome at later ages.

In our longitudinal study, 20 term and 20 preterm infants were assessed on the NBAS at three conceptual ages: 40 weeks, 42 weeks, and 44 weeks. Figure 3 shows the curves of two preterm infants. The preterm infant whose curve appears in 3A shows an optimal pattern of change, in our clinical judgment. The curve in 3B, also that of a preterm infant, indicates a change pattern that looks more worrisome.

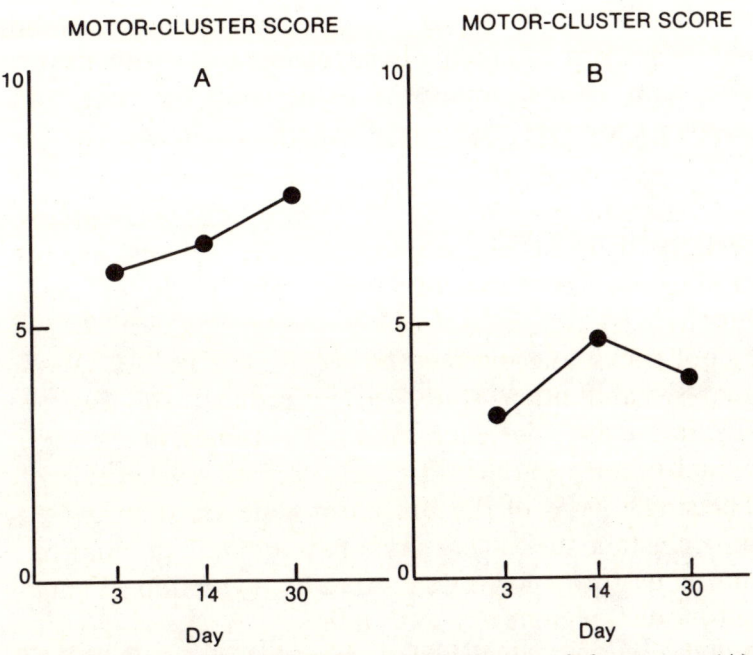

Figure 3. Motor-cluster curves of two preterm infants, one (A) showing an optimal pattern of change and one (B) a worrisome one. These curves predicted the infants' scores on the Bayley motor scale at 9 months with considerable accuracy.

LONGITUDINAL DATA. When the 40 infants in this study reached the age of 9 months, they were assessed on the Bayley Scales of Infant Development. Then their actual scores were compared with the scores we had predicted on the basis of the curve parameter scores. Although our findings need replication on larger samples before it will be appropriate to talk about statistical significance, some of our predictions were quite accurate, particularly those for the preterm group. For example, the correlation between the motor-cluster curve parameters and the Bayley Psychomotor Developmental Index scores for the preterm infants was .73. For the two preterm infants in Figure 3, we predicted Bayley motor scores of 131 for the infant in 3A and 84 for the infant in 3B. The actual scores were 134 and 87, respectively.

We also looked at the relationship between the Brazelton scale-curve parameter and the Infant Behavior Record that the examiner scores following the administration of the Bayley scales. We summarized the behavior record into five temperament-like dimensions and found strong relationships between the Brazelton curve parameters and the Bayley Scale for the baby's behavior at 9 months.

From early findings like these it appears that our method may be useful in relating the fluctuating behavior of newborn infants to later development. Our hope is that the patterns of change we have identified reflect continuity (if not stability) in newborn behavior. I would like to believe that they constitute a script describing the infant's adaptation to the postnatal environment, and that this script contains hints about the plot of the life story to come.

Brazelton: Now you see the kind of complexities we must get into if we're going to understand babies!

Carey: Barry, your project is basically an effort to cope with the fact that behaviors in the newborn have been found to be not very stable over time. But there may be other behaviors, different from the ones you've looked at, that would show more continuity — amount of motor activity, sensory threshold, and so on.

Lester: That's probably true. Our goal wasn't really to find behaviors that are stable. What we're interested in looking at, in fact, is the changes, because we think that the patterns of change reflect the coping capacities of the infant and will be our best predictor of future development.

Brazelton: Let me ask you all: When you begin to construct a model, don't you have to start with a clinician's a priori clustering? You can also do it statistically, with a computer, but I just wonder if it wouldn't be more economical to begin with clinical experience and then confirm it with the computer.

Bax: It does seem to me you might be better off starting with a qualitative analysis of the situation. I mean, it takes so much time to collect these data, and then when you're through the child isn't even a month old! I'm interested in them as they get older, too, and I think perhaps too much early analysis is going on here with not enough qualitative description of the whole pattern of the child's life.

Brazelton: I agree, Martin, that we in our lab are very hooked on that first month, and that we mustn't talk only about the neonate. But I think the same kinds of changes in patterns go on later, too, all the way through development.

McCall: I'm not trying to suggest that you replace thought with statistics, but I hope you all agree that the requirements for doing the statistics are ultimately the same as the requirements for clinical judgment; namely, you need a lot of experience with a lot of babies. Also, studies of adult thinking show that adults don't think in multivariate terms very often. We give some variables a lot of weight and ignore others. I think there's a danger of that happening when you're looking at a large multivariate system like infant behavior in a clinical situation, and one of the purposes of multivariate longitudinal statistics is to guard against it. The hope is that the procedures, used appropriately, will help get rid of prejudice and error.

Taft: Still, statistical gymnastics turn a lot of people off. Some clinicians just don't want to look at behavior in terms of numbers.

Brazelton: I hear what you're saying, and I agree. But as clinicians many of us need documentation that we can use in our own minds to support our so-called clinical intuition. The field of neonatal assessment started with nurses' "intuitions" that this was a good premie or a bad one, a good baby or a bad one. But it wasn't really intuition at all — it was a computer just like Barry's. So I think, if we study these things statistically, then we can back people up and say, go ahead with your eyes and your hands and your working with people, and believe in it.

Denhoff: Barry, speaking as a pediatrician in the office every day, I would say you have given me enough information to alert me to some clusters of behavior. You've given us something to look at, and that is a start.

Assessing Infant Individuality

by Heidelise Als, Ph.D.

The Assessment of Preterm Infants' Behavior (APIB), developed by Heidelise Als and her colleagues, is a modification of the Brazelton Neonatal Behavioral Assessment Scale (NBAS) for use with preterm infants. Like the NBAS, the APIB consists of a series of interactions between the examiner and the newborn. Both tests are customarily administered while parents look on, and the examiner often comments or "interprets" while putting the infant through his or her paces. After watching an assessment, parents often handle their baby more skillfully and with greater confidence. As Brazelton puts it in his Introduction, "Each assessment in which parents participate does automatically become an intervention."

In her paper, Als explains how the NBAS and the APIB can be used to study infant individuality. Newborns differ, for example, in the strategies they use to calm themselves. They also differ in their ability to organize their behavior and reach their behavioral goals efficiently. Als' work suggests that such differences are not short-lived but remain at least until the age of 9 months.

While the infant researcher strives to uncover patterns and regularities, usually by studying homogeneous groups of subjects, the parent and the clinician are confronted with individual infants. Our work is aimed at uncovering patterns and regularities that will allow the adults who deal with infants to understand and support their individuality.

I first became interested in assessing individuality when I started as a school teacher in Germany. My first teaching assignment was a classroom of 28 third-graders. Although I thought I was quite well prepared for my job, I did not anticipate the large individual differences that I saw in the responses of children of similar intellectual competence to the teaching and learning situation.

My memory of two children is especially vivid. The first was Reinhardt, who always arrived at least half an hour before class started. Looking wide-eyed and very tense, he would march past my desk, sit down in the first row, and set out all his implements. Ten minutes before class started, he was completely ready to learn. The second child was Wolfgang. Just before the bell rang, he would saunter to his seat at the back of the room, perhaps telling me a little joke as he passed. He always had a hidden comic book, which of course was not allowed, and he loved to play pranks on the children and me. But he did his work beautifully.

Despite the similarity of their report cards, these children were very different. For one, life seemed a sequence of opportunities to thrive on and enjoy; for the other, it was a sequence of costly onslaughts to be coped with. Wherein lies the difference? How can we, as researchers, tap the expandability or costliness of the organism's efforts as it negotiates its developmental agenda?

In our work with newborns, we have been using the Brazelton Neonatal Behavioral Assessment Scale (NBAS) and a modification of it that we developed, called the Assessment of Preterm Infants' Behavior (APIB), to assess differences in infants' capacities for regulating and integrating their behavior. When an examiner administers these scales, she or he essentially plays the role of structurer and organizer of the infant's environment. As the examiner brings the baby from sleep to alert to crying states and back down to calm alertness, she or he presents the infant with packages of increasingly demanding environmental inputs. How does the infant cope with these? What adaptive strategies does the baby use, how smoothly, and at what expense?

One of our early findings will serve to illustrate. Underweight infants born at term, we discovered, tend to have more difficulty than average-weight infants in attaining the calm, expansive, alert state required for interaction with the examiner. Even at ten days of age, an underweight's transition from sleep to alertness was likely to be "expensive," accompanied by many signs of effort and stress, such as clenched fists (or splayed fingers), tension (or limpness) of the arms and legs, pallor around the mouth, and perhaps hiccoughing, a bowel movement, or even spitting up.

NEWBORN SELF-REGULATING STRATEGIES. Although there are various ways for an examiner to help smooth an infant's behavior, we began to understand that infants themselves, at each stage of their development, have balancing and integration strategies that allow them to return to balance on their own. These

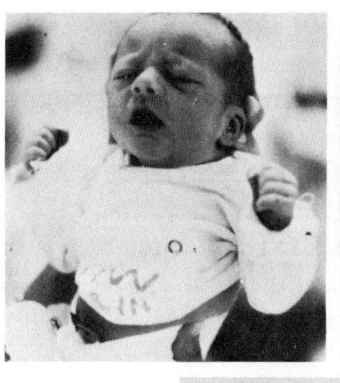

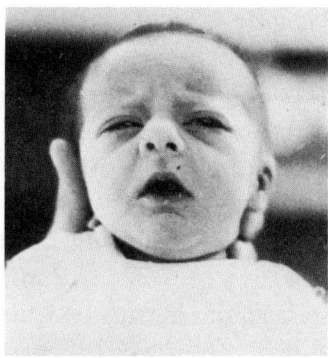

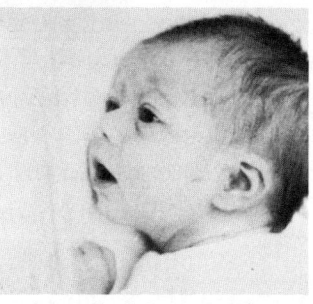

Figure 4. As the strained facial expression and clenched hands show, reaching an alert state entails considerable effort and cost for this underweight newborn. From H. Als, E. Tronick, L. Adamson, and T. B. Brazelton, The Behavior of the fullterm but underweight newborn infant. *Developmental Medicine and Child Neurology* **18**:590-602. 1976. Reproduced with permission.

strategies may be quite sophisticated (such as yawning) or quite primitive (such as tremor). If the infant is stressed too much, balance will be difficult to achieve.

When we started to work with preterm infants, these issues became even more obvious. In a pilot study comparing the behavior of ten preterm and ten term infants at the same post-conceptual age, we found the preterms to be more sensitive to environmental inputs, more easily stressed and overstimulated, and more likely to overreact. They seemed to need more finely tuned environmental structuring and support than the term infants in order to free up their best performance on our test items. Their individual capacities, such as visual tracking, were often as good as those of the term infants, but the organization of their behavior was consistently different.

Despite the small size of our sample, we were able to identify four distinct groups or clusters of infants. The clusters differed in motor capacity, attentional capacity, and mean organizational capacity, and they could be ranked from most well organized to least well organized. The infants in Cluster 1, the best-organized group, showed well-developed behavior in all three categories. The babies in Cluster 2 did somewhat less well in all three, and the babies in Cluster 4 did poorly in all three. Cluster 3 is perhaps the most interesting, because it was characterized by good motor and overall organizational capacities but very poor attentional capacity. These clusters cut across the medical variables of birth weight and gestational age, though there was some tendency for preterm infants to fall into the lower groups.

OLDER INFANTS. Our next question was, do these clusters relate to later functioning? As a first step toward an answer, we examined the same 20 infants after they had reached the age of 9 months. The conceptual issues in the later study were the same as in the earlier one. In the face of comparable skill development (as assessed on the Bayley scales, for instance), are there differences in children's strategies for organization and self-regulation that we can assess? Can we identify the newly emerging developmental agenda at this age?

We observed the infants in a structured play situation, both alone and in cooperation with a parent. Once again, an analysis of the scores revealed four naturally occurring clusters that differed along dimensions of organizational capacity and could be ranked according to "goodness." Further, most of the 9-month-old infants belonged to a cluster whose rank was the same as or adjacent to the rank of the cluster each had belonged to as a newborn.

Although the particular configurations of behavior that we have identified are tentative, pending research with larger samples, our general approach has already benefited many families. The conceptual model of a total organism, constantly bringing the skills it has available to bear on its environment and trying to make the world work for it, offers a framework within which parents and other caregivers can understand the specific dynamics, needs, sensitivities, and strengths of an infant. It helps them sharpen their observations, and use them to modify their input and provide structure for the baby. It encourages sensitivity to the infant's current developmental agenda and teaches parents ways of fostering the increasing autonomy, richness, flexibility, and self-regulation of their infants.

Denhoff: Your work calls into question the common belief that 2000- or 1500-gram babies recover quite well, becoming perfectly normal by around 2 or 3 years. Physically normal and mentally normal, yes, but I wonder about attentional capacity, for example. There may be differences in individual outcome for this preterm group that we have overlooked.

Als: The integration of physical well-being, and of skills, is where some of our preterm babies seem to have more trouble than babies with different starts. Still, there are babies with medically good starts who face similar organizational issues, and in our group of preterm babies some were quite well regulated. What I'm proposing is that the behavior of the baby can tell us what that baby's issues and difficulties are.

McCall: That would be very useful information to share with parents.

Als: I agree. Mothers have a range of expectancies about infant behavior, and if their own child's behavior isn't within that range, the mother may need to make a conscious and deliberate accommodation to the child. Premies, difficult babies, babies with sensory defects and so on often demand that the environment expand what it "normally" does, and the baby's little behavioral signals show just what works well for that particular child.

Brazelton: One of the things that struck me, as an

observer, was how closely parents manage to identify with their baby while watching Heidi's exam. This can be a powerful process.

Taft: Heidi, I have two questions. First, you said that a preterm baby, born at 34 weeks and tested six weeks later, still did not have the self-regulatory patterns of a 40-week term infant tested at birth. Can you speculate why? What difference does the extrauterine environment make as compared with the intrauterine environment? Second, how well did your mothers do at learning to deal with the infant's behavior? Do you think your instruction really made a difference?

Als: When an infant is born before term, organ systems that are structured to be facilitated by the mother's body are prematurely required to act on their own. The respiratory system, for instance, has to get going, and we use a lot of medical support to get it going. I'm speculating, but I feel there's an internal discrepancy in the readiness of the systems that are called on to start functioning, quite apart from environmental differences before and after birth. Future studies of normal fetal development will teach us to create extrauterine environments that are more appropriate to the nervous system, I hope.

As for your second question, we need to remember that the mother of an infant born early is also premature. She hasn't gone through the usual final phases of preparation. Nevertheless, we haven't found a mother yet who wasn't ready to put tremendous energy into nurturing this baby. Often, the mother has learned a great deal about the child but lacks confidence. She doesn't give herself credit for interpreting the baby's signs correctly. So we give her license to take her own reactions seriously. We help her see her baby and herself as individuals instead of always looking for general rules.

Bax: Statements about "giving the mother license" make me uneasy. Most babies of most mothers, small or not, don't do very well on their own. Perhaps we should just leave the mother alone to go on with her baby and not be so quick to nudge in.

Parmelee: Still, in clinical practice we do meet some mothers who disappoint us in their way of handling babies. You can't leave all of them alone and expect them to do well. I think this suggests we may need to get *more* involved, for instance by training teenagers in the facts of mothering.

Als: We don't want to add just another prescription for mothers to follow, but I think the baby's behavior is a safeguard against that. In focusing our attention on this baby's way of handling environmental requirements, we are fostering the mother's confidence in the baby's cues and her own ability to read them.

Toward a Model of Early Infant Development

by Frances Degen Horowitz, Ph.D.

Frances Horowitz is firmly opposed to explanations of human development that are based only on characteristics of infants or only on characteristics of their environments. Variables of both types are important, and the challenge is to discover how they interact. In "Toward a Model of Early Infant Development," Horowitz reviews research attempting to relate infant behavior, as assessed on a modification of the Brazelton Neonatal Behavioral Assessment Scale (NBAS) called the NBAS-K, to independent observations of infant-mother interaction.

Two studies that Horowitz describes included only lower-class mother-infant pairs. In the discussion following her paper, Horowitz suggests that replication with a middle-class sample might yield different findings. From this point in the conference on, the effects of socioeconomic status on infant development received increasing amounts of attention from the participants.

An evaluation of only the infant or only the environment will never net us an understanding of human development, which is probably the most complex phenomenon on this planet. An accurate model of development must include variables associated with the organism as well as variables associated with the environment, and it should depict developmental outcome as resulting from interactions within and across these domains.

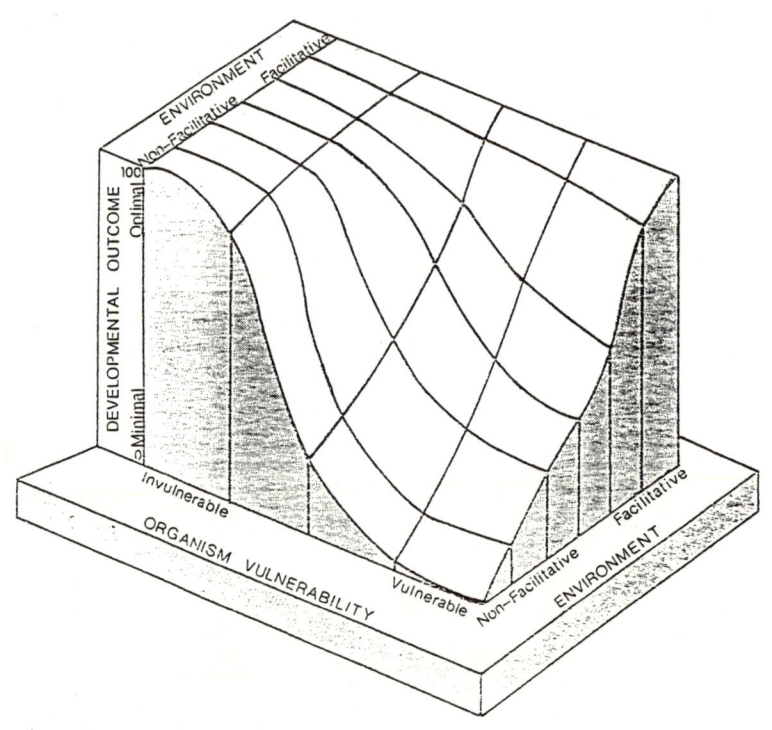

Figure 5. A three-dimensional model of organism-environment relationships and developmental outcome.

An attempt at such a model appears in Figure 5. Its top surface describes the adequacy of developmental outcome, which is determined by the interaction between organismic vulnerability on the one hand and environmental facilitation or nonfacilitation on the other. Since qualities of the organism and the environment can change as time passes, a relatively poor developmental outcome may give way to a better one, or vice versa. For example, a child who is relatively invulnerable to outside influences during infancy — a very self-sufficient baby, so to speak — might become a less invulnerable preschooler, and thus depend more heavily on favorable environmental factors for best development during that period.

Such a model can help reorient the issues surrounding continuity and discontinuity in development. Continuity will be demonstrated across developmental periods as long as the values of the functional variables do not show significant change; discontinuity will be found where the values do show major change.

NATURE-NURTURE CONTROVERSY. The model also helps in the refocusing of the nature-nurture controversy. Traditionally, there are two extremes on the nativist-empiricist continuum. At the nativist end, exemplified by Descartes, is the belief that the growth and development of a human being is largely predetermined by heredity. In this view, a basically benign and supportive environment ensures the natural unfolding of the organism's behavioral repertoire. At the other end, exemplified by Locke, is the empiricist view of the human newborn as a "white paper, devoid of characters and without any ideas" (Locke 1690) until written upon by systematic encounters with experience.

An "either/or" approach to questions of heredity and environment pits these extremes against each other. The more current approach, in contrast, is an interactional one. Nature can be viewed as playing a strong role in the newborn's behavioral repertoire, in later behavior that depends on the biological system, and in the organism's level of sensitivity to environmental impact. Nurture can be seen as having a strong role in what stimulation is available to the child, whether it is appropriate to the child's developmental level, and so on. The task of the behavioral scientist is to discover the laws that govern interactions between these variables.

The Brazelton Neonatal Behavioral Assessment Scale (NBAS) has been an important tool in our attempt to understand how an infant's characteristics interact with environmental stimulation. Because of the particular goals of our research at the University of Kansas, we have modified the NBAS in two ways. First, we made provision for scoring infants' modal behavior as well as their best performance, since we planned to try to relate their scores to interactions with their mothers rather than with highly trained Brazelton examiners. Second, we added five scale items: orientation to inanimate visual and auditory stimulus (a rattle), quality of infant's alert responsivity, infant's general irritability, examiner's persistence (how hard the examiner had to work to elicit the scored behavior), and reinforcement value of the infant's behavior (essentially, how much the examiner liked the infant). The modified scale is referred to as the NBAS-K.

INFANT-MOTHER INTERACTION. Much of our work so far has been directed at obtaining NBAS-K scores for newborns that we can then relate to independent observations of infant-environment interactions. In a study of infant-mother interactions during the newborn period, Linn evaluated 28 infants born to low socioeconomic-status (SES) mothers, administering the NBAS-K at two days and three days of age. In addition, two independent half-hour observations were made of mother and infant during feeding sessions at the hospital. An extensive observational code was devised to record the infant's behavior, the mother's behavior, and stimuli in the environmental surroundings.

We expected to find that infants who showed more stable behavior on the two NBAS-K exams would have mothers whose behavior was more responsive. A simple line of reasoning influenced this conjecture — the mother of an infant exhibiting a stable repertoire of behavior knows what to expect and thus should be better prepared to respond. As things turned out, the opposite was true. Infants whose behavior was *variable* tended to be involved in interactions with mothers who were more responsive.

This finding has strengthened our suspicion that variability is an inherent characteristic of early infant behavior, an informative parameter rather than a nuisance. A certain degree of infant variability may be evolutionarily adaptive, giving the infant a greater chance to respond to changing environmental contexts. Variability may also stimulate caregiving behavior by holding the caregiver's attention and interest.

Twenty of the infants Linn tested at the hospital were tested again by Buddin at two weeks and one month of age. The NBAS-K was administered at both ages. At one month, two 4-hour home observations were also made, using the same extensive observational code as before.

At one month, we found a strong and consistent relationship between the infant's performance on the Brazelton orientation items and one aspect of maternal caregiving. In general, the lower the infant's modal orientation scores, the more cuddling and holding on the part of the mother. In other words, for these low SES mother-infant pairs, infants with lower orientation performance on the modified Brazelton exam received more enveloping tactile stimulation from their mothers. Further, when Buddin categorized the mothers in her sample as generally responsive or unresponsive, she found that more stable infant behavior on two NBAS-K exams predicted *unresponsive* behavior in the mother.

These results were unexpected, and they raise many questions. Are the patterns we have observed in the first days of life and again at one month particular to a lower socioeconomic group? If so, we can see some possible very early sources of the patterns of development typically associated with lower SES children. We are now replicating Buddin's and Linn's work with middle-class mother-infant pairs in order to determine if the same relationships obtain.

HIGH-RISK INFANTS. Our efforts to study the environmental experience and interactional patterns of high-risk infants have just begun. We have done some work with infants with very mild risk conditions and some with infants whose risk status is more severe.

A mild risk condition whose developmental sequelae are not entirely understood involves slightly to moderately elevated bilirubin levels in the first days of life. The standard treatment in American hospitals is to place such infants under bilirubin lights as a form of phototherapy. Phototherapy is demonstrably effective in reducing bilirubin levels, but the possible effects on behavioral and other development have just begun to be documented.

Nelson used the NBAS-K to compare the behavior of a group of infants just before phototherapy with that of a matched comparison sample of infants not needing phototherapy. Both groups were assessed three more times: just after termination of phototherapy, at two weeks, and at one month of age. Though there were few significant differences between the groups, an interesting consistency emerged in the data. Right after treatment and at two weeks of age, the treated infants generally showed poorer performance than the comparison infants. Only about half the infants could be followed up at one month of age, but the trend held then as well. However, the differences between groups were not large and may have no functional significance.

We are also concerned with more seriously at-risk infants, such as those born prematurely who spend considerable time in a neonatal intensive care unit. Because we want to obtain comparable data from preterm and term infants, our first task has been to determine whether the NBAS-K can be used with preterms. Dailey's work with 30 preterm infants indicates that it can, supplemented with some qualifying observations.

Dailey's most intriguing finding should be mentioned. Infants whose behavior at 1800 grams appeared to be stronger (babies who were, for example, less tremulous, more consolable, and higher in reinforcement value) had discharge weights a week to ten days later that were higher than the discharge weights of the other babies. We do not entirely understand this relationship, since one might expect that an infant with more "put-together" behavior would be discharged at a somewhat *lower* weight.

The program of research I have described seems to confirm that studying only infant characteristics and not those of the functional environment or vice versa will never yield an accurate map of behavioral development. From our data and that of others, it appears that individual differences at birth may have important influences on how the environment responds to newborn infants and on how much impact, positive or negative, environmental factors are likely to have. The caregiving skills of primary caretakers are also important contributors to infant-environment interactions. If our data hold and our theoretical speculations are supported, it may become possible to identify infant-caretaker-environment combinations that permit us to predict different developmental outcomes and to hone our intervention techniques to specific problems.

McCall: Frances, would your findings be consistent with something like this? In order to have an interaction, there has to be a certain amount of behavior going on, and if the baby is doing a lot of it, the mother doesn't need to do so much. If the baby is lethargic for one reason or another, the mother has to make up for this and be more active in trying to elicit behavior from the infant. Would that be a possible explanation for some of the things you're observing?

Horowitz: Yes, except that my prediction is we're not going to find the same patterns in the middle class. I could be wrong, of course.

Brazelton: In your studies of term infants, both samples were lower class?

Horowitz: Yes, all lower-class, black mothers, many of them single parents. We're collecting data on a middle-class sample now.

Als: I looked at a very small sample of middle-class

babies in England, and it did seem that the lethargic baby got jazzing-up input and the irritable baby got soothing-down input. It was as if the environment was geared to support the baby to a certain level and then let him do his own thing, if you will. It would be interesting to look at the inputs he elicits then.

Horowitz: We need to identify the characteristics of facilitative environments for infants. They may not be identical for all social classes.

McCall: In my paper I'll be making the point that socioeconomic status seems to predict later outcome for a child as well as or better than anything else. But it isn't clear just what socioeconomic status means. It's a marker variable, not a functional variable.

Parmelee: One thing socioeconomic status does is put some constraints on the shifts in the environment that occur with time. When we describe a child's environment, we describe it at a particular moment in time. A year later, it might be very different. The child might have a different caretaker or a completely reorganized family. We need to add changes in the time dimension to our model of development.

Carey: Something else one should consider is the things we physicians do that affect parent-child interaction in the newborn period. Our own behavior is an "environmental factor" we often overlook. For instance, physiological jaundice, which is the usual reason the bilirubin light is used in the hospital nursery, is probably a variation of normal up to a moderate degree, but some pediatricians regard it as always a disease. It seems to me that the more the pediatrician thinks of it as a disease, the more likely he or she will be to use the bilirubin light — and also to communicate this anxiety to the parents. Surely this concern will influence their interactions with their babies. Theoretically, failure to consider the physician's role in the interaction gives an inadequate view of the situation. From a practical point of view, I think the lesson is that pediatricians should take care not to worry parents needlessly.

Lubchenco: With jaundice, the anxiety one produces may be warranted. Until you get some measure of unbound bilirubin, you are going to worry.

Carey: If the bilirubin level is high enough, we all begin to worry.

Lubchenco: It's not necessarily high, though — that's the catch. What I'm thinking of is the study I talked about earlier, in which the babies with physiological jaundice did worse later on than the ones with higher bilirubin levels. I had to express my concern, because this is a real problem.

Barnard: Did the infants have other metabolic problems?

Lubchenco: No, these babies were slightly preterm infants who did not have a lot of other problems.

Carey: Well, remember you are talking about infants in a controlled study run at a teaching hospital. In the community hospitals that I'm more familiar with, I think you'll find that the bilirubin lights tend to go on earlier and stay on longer. The decision isn't always made with the degree of care that you see in teaching hospitals. There is considerable overtreatment and consequently many parents are given the impression that their babies are sicker than they really are.

Horowitz: We've found a little support for that idea. One of the pediatricians we worked with said he hadn't realized he was putting babies under the lights when their bilirubin levels were so low, down around 10 or 11.

McCall: Fran, your work and the work discussed in the two papers before yours have shown us some interesting uses of an infant test that does not have one of the characteristics frequently used to judge tests, namely predictability. The Brazelton scale has been accused not only of not predicting down the road but maybe of not predicting even five days from now! Yet, as we've seen, it is a good index of contemporary status, and the status of the baby offers clues as to how the parent will interact with the child at that time. The test can also be used to tell us about the qualitative nature of developmental change, if you use the items in that way rather than simply looking at total scores.

Neurophysiological Assessment of the Neonate
by Frank H. Duffy, M.D.

Frank Duffy's presentation was by far the most visually exciting of our round table. Duffy showed videotapes, in full color, of a new technique for neurophysiological assessment called BEAM, for Brain Electrical Activity Mapping. The technique improves the visibility of electroencephalographic and evoked-potential data by transforming numbers into visual images like those shown in Figure 6.

Using BEAM and other techniques, Duffy and his coworkers have distinguished between normal newborns and newborns who are probably (though not obviously) abnormal, and also between normal and dyslexic boys of school age. Duffy's findings on dyslexia suggest that it involves abnormal functioning in a considerably larger portion of the brain than is generally supposed.

Advances in medical technology have brought remarkable improvements in the mortality rate of prematurely born infants. As a result, physicians find themselves increasingly responsible for providing a suitable extrauterine environment for these tiny babies. For optimum development, should that environment be made protective and womb-like, stimulating and increasingly complex, or doesn't it matter? Possibly the course of neuro-behavioral development is fixed by the genes, and the environment plays a role only in extreme situations.

These considerations assume additional importance with the mounting evidence that small preterm infants are overrepresented in the population of learning-disabled school children. Drillien and her colleagues have demonstrated that approximately 50% of small-for-gestational-age preterm infants experience some school-related difficulty. What role does the environment play in determining which 50% do well and which not so well? If we could identify the 50% maximally at risk, could we prevent risk from becoming reality?

For these questions to be pursued, two key elements must fall into place. First, there must be definitive evidence demonstrating that the environment has a significant impact on neuro-behavioral development. Second, there must be sensitive and quantitative methodologies for identifying the group at greatest risk and for assessing the effects of a changed environment on that group.

BRAIN CELLS AND ENVIRONMENT IN KITTENS. Hubel and Wiesel's classic experiments on the visual system of the cat demonstrate a definite interaction between the environment and brain development. If one of a newborn kitten's eyes is sutured closed at birth and kept closed for several months, the animal appears blind in the eye when it is later opened and tested. Further, stimulating the eye does not activate any cortical cells. These visual deficiencies are relatively permanent. Since prolonged deprivation in an adult cat has no significant effect, Hubel and Wiesel have proposed a critical period during which manipulations of the visual environment can profoundly affect neural development. In the kitten, this period runs from 4 to 16 weeks of age. More subtle restrictions of the visual environment have also been shown to modify vision, but only during comparable critical periods.

It is interesting that these findings can be used to bolster opposing viewpoints toward intervention. From one perspective, the work is an affirmation of the profound effect of the environment upon the development of brain and behavior. Those with this perspective see supportive measures and intervention as potentially very beneficial. The other perspective emphasizes the extreme nature of the environmental manipulations necessary to produce an effect. It stresses the stability of brain and behavior outside the critical period and the difficulty of defining the bounds of such a period in human infants. This view minimizes environmental influences and sees little promise in early intervention.

More recent animal work in our laboratory seems to support the first of these positions. Our studies show, first, that the brain is not necessarily immutable beyond the critical period, and second, that the timing of the critical period itself can be influenced by environmental events.

These findings may have a direct parallel in preterm human infants. Perhaps premature exposure to the complex stimuli of the world outside the womb triggers a critical (or at least sensitive) period that the immature preterm infant cannot fully take advantage of. Behavioral evidence suggests that premature infants actively withdraw from or shut out stimuli that full-term infants handle with relative ease. If premature infants are partially deprived during a sensitive period, this could contribute to the sensory-motor and learning problems many of them show as they grow older.

Animal experimentation has brought this and other provocative possibilities to mind. However, animal studies cannot provide definitive answers to questions about human infants.

METHODOLOGIES FOR HUMAN ASSESSMENT. Our approach to infant assessment uses instruments from three quite different methodological areas: infant behavioral assessment, neurophysiology, and automated classification statistics.

1. Infant behavioral assessment: Assessment of Preterm Infant Behavior (APIB).

The APIB, developed by Als and her colleagues, is a modification of the Brazelton Neonatal Behavioral Assessment Scale for use with preterm infants. As Als explains in her paper, p. 26, the APIB provides a behavioral profile that reflects the infant's capacity for organizing and integrating his or her behavior.

2. Neurophysiological assessment: Brain Electrical Activity Mapping (BEAM) and Significance Probability Mapping (SPM).

Electroencephalography (EEG) and sensory evoked potentials (EP) are established clinical methods for neurological evaluation. Over the last several years, we have developed a simple yet effective means of improving the visibility of EEG and EP data by means of computerized topographic mapping. We call our procedure Brain Electrical Activity Mapping or BEAM.

Significance Probability Mapping (SPM) represents an extension of BEAM. It addresses the question of how, when one examines a BEAM image, one can determine what topographic regions are normal or abnormal. The goal is to make visible characteristics of the data that otherwise might not be evident. This requires a statistical-to-optical transformation. The numerical data that underlie the original BEAM image undergo statistical manipulation. The results are themselves transformed into an image, which is then presented within the coordinate system or framework of the original data. SPM can be used to delineate regions of difference between two BEAM images, as shown in Figure 6.

To assess the usefulness of BEAM and SPM, we undertook a study comparing the brain activity of eight dyslexic and 10 normal boys, aged 9 to 11 years. Community surveys have shown that dyslexia affects 3.5 to 6% of school-age children. Sixty percent of all children referred to the Learning Disabilities Clinic at Children's Hospital Medical Center, Boston, have a measurable degree of reading disability.

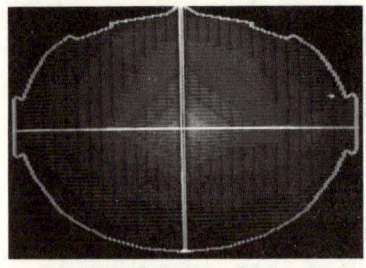

A. BEAM plot, Group 1 (normal)

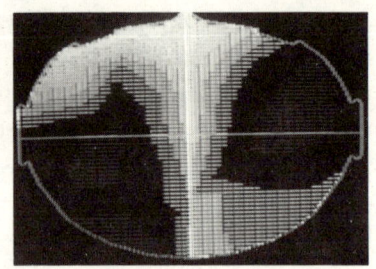

B. BEAM plot, Group 2 (probably abnormal)

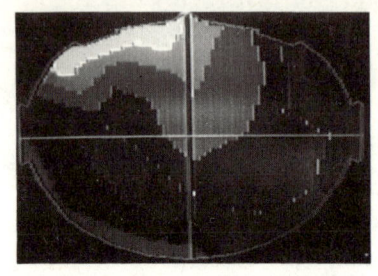

C. Significance Probability Map (SPM) showing regions of difference between Groups 1 and 2

Figure 6. This figure illustrates the formation of a Significance Probability Map (SPM) to answer the question, Where do Groups 1 and 2 differ in EEG delta activity? The SPM in C shows that the two groups differ in delta in the frontal lobes, left greater than right.

The evidence we obtained suggests that the physiological aberrations in the brains of dyslexics are more widespread than was previously suspected. EEG and EP data were recorded during behavioral testing of each boy on a variety of tasks. Analysis by BEAM and SPM revealed several discrete regions of difference between the dyslexic and normal groups: (1) the classic speech region, encompassing the left midtemporal lobe and left posterior quadrant, (2) the left antero-lateral frontal region, and (3) a large bilateral medial frontal-lobe area.

Concurrent work in Scandinavia using another methodology has demonstrated that these same regions are activated in normal people by speech, reading silently, and reading aloud. In other words, the regions normally active in linguistic tasks were the regions identified through BEAM and SPM as differing between dyslexics and normals. We concluded that dyslexia represents a dysfunction of the entire cortical system normally engaged in speech and reading rather than an isolated lesion, as might be predicted by analogy with aphasia in adults.

3. Automated classification statistics: TICAS.

"Automated classification" refers to the branch of statistics that deals with the development and testing of diagnostic rules. It is accomplished in the same way that clinicians come to recognize and diagnose (or classify) illness, though by computer. When faced with a population of patients having a previously undescribed illness, clinicians obtain a number of measurements on each patient (such as temperature, vital signs, presence of a rash). Next they search for those measurements most descriptive and specific for this disease. They formulate a diagnostic rule based on those features and test it by seeing how well it diagnoses or classifies new patients suspected of having this new disease. Automated classification procedures follow essentially the same steps.

Although it was developed for the automated identification of malignant cells from digitized images (a task in which its success has been remarkable), the TICAS system for automated classification can be readily used in other ways. We have used TICAS to analyze neurophysiological data and formulate diagnostic rules that (1) discriminate workers with histories of organophosphate exposure from nonexposed workers, and (2) discriminate children with dyslexia from normal children.

PILOT STUDY WITH NEONATES. As mentioned earlier, some 50% of infants born very early and below expected gestational weight will encounter learning difficulties — and 50% will not. Might the methodologies just outlined make it possible to predict in early infancy which infants will fall into which group?

In our pilot work in this area, 11 neonates were selected for combined behavioral and neurophysiological investigation. All were considered normal by their physicians. However, clustering procedures and diagnostic rules developed in earlier work with the APIB and TICAS indicated that six infants were likely to be less competent than the other five. We called this group of six the PROB group. The five infants who seemed more competent were called the NICE group.

Both groups were studied extensively in the neurophysiology lab. The following observations were made:
  (1) BEAM and classic EEG showed more difference in brain activity during a change in behavioral state for group NICE than for group PROB.
  (2) BEAM with SPM identified regional differences in brain activity between the two groups in the frontal, temporal, and occipital lobes.
  (3) Sleep EEG demonstrated more "premature" patterns in group PROB than in group NICE.

These data suggest that behavioral clustering can be expected to have correlates in measures of brain electrical activity. Moreover, topographic displays assist in the localization of functional differences between behavioral clusters.

These results, though preliminary, are encouraging. We hope that refinements of our combined methodology will not only permit more accurate and meaningful assessment of infant neuro-behavioral organization but provide outcome measures for testing developmental hypotheses generated by animal experimentation.

McCall: How do you interpret the neurological differences between your two groups of infants, Frank? Would you speculate on that?

Duffy: Well, speaking speculatively, it seemed to me the differences might be telling us something about the functioning of higher associative cortex in the two groups. In my view, what the associative cortex does is to permit the kind of cross-modal associations that make human problem solvers say "Oh yes, I see!" Chimps can do this too — make mental connections, put two things together — but rhesus monkeys and other lower primates cannot. So it is intuitively appealing to me that a less competent organism might have different function in this region, or might have to use more different regions to get the same net performance.

McCall: Would you offer the same interpretation of the mappings of the dyslexic boys in your earlier studies — more isolated learning and less cross-modal transferring?

Duffy: Let's suppose that we had determined that these dyslexic children, now age 25 and all able to read, still had the same brain patterns. My speculation would be that they had a different brain organization, one that today's society selects out as less desirable. Years ago, a fellow who maybe wasn't very good at speech might have had some other genetic advantage.

Parmelee: Maybe there are lots of slightly different brain organizations, and this one happens to make it harder to do what today's society requires at age 6, which is to read.

Brazelton: I think Frank's studies encourage us to look at the neurological process as a whole rather than just in terms of a stimulus and a response, which is the way we've looked at neurological function for too long. It seems to me Frank has shown that there are differences in the ways babies and children process information, and that these differences relate to their failure or success.

Denhoff: Have you looked at any adults who used to be dyslexic but have apparently recovered?

Duffy: A prejudice of mine is that I don't think dyslexics do recover. I think they learn to read and function very well, but they often return for medical assistance when they can't pass the language requirements for a Ph.D., or they go into professions where reading skills don't need to be highly developed. We're recruiting subjects for a study now from a local college of art and a local college of engineering, where we think there may be a lot of successful but rather inarticulate students with family histories of dyslexia.

Brazelton: When you talk about a kind of fixation or rigidity of the system in children with problems, it seems to me that you're talking about a cost-effective system within the baby or child that includes not only differences in the ways children process information but differences in the way they adapt to the environment. Perhaps economy and fixation typify the child who has problems whereas a broad, more adaptive scanning system is more normal. I think this may be where we'll have to head before we're through.

Early Screening for Developmental Delays and Potential School Problems
by William K. Frankenburg, M.D.

William Frankenburg's description of new work with a classic screening instrument, the Denver Developmental Screening Test (DDST), returns us to the fascinating topics of social class and home environment. Developed by Frankenburg and Dodds, the DDST has been used to screen thousands of preschool children for developmental deficits since its publication in 1967.

Recently, a short test was developed for use before the full DDST. A prescreen, it was thought, would make screening on a large scale even more practical. Selected DDST items were rewritten as a questionnaire to be answered by parents, and this prescreen was found to identify middle-class children with deficits. It was less successful with lower SES populations. For the latter, a prescreen consisting of selected DDST items administered by an examiner has been devised and works well.

The second innovation Frankenburg describes is a questionnaire about home environment, based on Bettye Caldwell's well-known Inventory of Home Stimulation (STIM) and developed with her assistance. Frankenburg and his coworkers are currently evaluating the ability of this questionnaire, used in conjunction with the DDST, to identify preschool children who will probably have achievement problems after they enter school. In poverty populations, this group may include as many as 50% of all children.

For the past 15 years, my colleagues and I have been involved in developing screening procedures for early identification of developmental delays. More recently, we have turned our attention to screening for potential school problems, especially among children in lower socioeconomic groups. The rate of school achievement problems in children from disadvantaged environments is approximately 50%. Many of these problems can be alleviated if the children are identified early and referred for appropriate intervention.

SCREENING FOR DEVELOPMENTAL DELAYS: THE DDST AND THE PDQ. Screening, as defined by the United States Commission on Chronic Illness and by the World Health Organization, involves the use of quick, easily administered procedures with an asymptomatic population in order to differentiate individuals who probably have the condition in question from those who do not. Screening tests are not diagnostic; they merely identify some people as suspect. A diagnostic evaluation must then be done to determine whether a person has the condition being screened for.

Our screening procedures are designed for use with children between birth and 6 years of age. Our first test, the Denver Developmental Screening Test (DDST), appeared in 1967. It was standardized on 1,036 presumably normal children, 2 weeks to 6 years old, whose families reflect the ethnic and occupational population of Denver.

The DDST consists of 105 items arranged in four categories of functioning: personal-social, fine motor-adaptive, language, and gross motor. Equipment needs are minimal: small blocks, a tennis ball, a skein of wool, and a few other simple materials. To administer the test, approximately 20 age-appropriate items (that is, items passed by 90% of children in the normative sample) are given. The child's score is then classified as normal, abnormal, questionable (borderline) or untestable. All children who receive other than normal results should be retested one week later to rule out temporary effects such as illness, hunger, fatigue, and fear caused by separation from the parent.

The test has widespread acceptance in the professional community and has been translated into numerous foreign languages. It has almost universal appeal to children, since they view it as a game. Parents generally enjoy the test because their children enjoy it, and because they are anxious to see what the child will do with the developmental tasks. Administration of the DDST is easy for anyone who enjoys playing with young children, provided he or she can read at a seventh-grade level and studies the manual.

Reliability studies show that the DDST, though administered by nonprofessionals, generates tester-observer and test-retest reliabilities comparable to those of longer diagnostic tests administered by psychologists, such as the Bayley Scales of Infant Development. Its validity is also high. For example, in a study comparing children's DDST scores with their scores on the revised Bayley Infant Scales (for children under 2) or the Stanford-Binet (for children 2 and over), the DDST identified 92% of children with developmental quotients below 70 and 97% of the children with DQs or IQs of 70 and above.

With the banning of IQ tests in some schools and related concern over racial discrimination, the question of whether some developmental screening tests are inappropriate for certain segments of the population has been raised. A recent study has shed light on this matter. The study compared the DDST scores of 1,055 lower-class infants and preschoolers (349 Anglo, 352 black, and 354 Spanish-surname children of unskilled workers) with the scores of 1,180 children representing a cross-section of Denver's ethnic and parental-occupation groups. Below 20 months of age, we found, infants from the unskilled sample were developmentally advanced over infants from the cross-sectional sample, which was mainly middle class. After 20 months of age, children in the cross-sectional sample were more advanced, except in the personal-social category. Comparisons of Anglo, black, and Spanish-surname children in the unskilled sample revealed few differences. These findings suggest that socioeconomic status (rather than ethnicity) accounts for differences in development, that the differences appear by 20 months of age, and that the DDST is not racially biased.

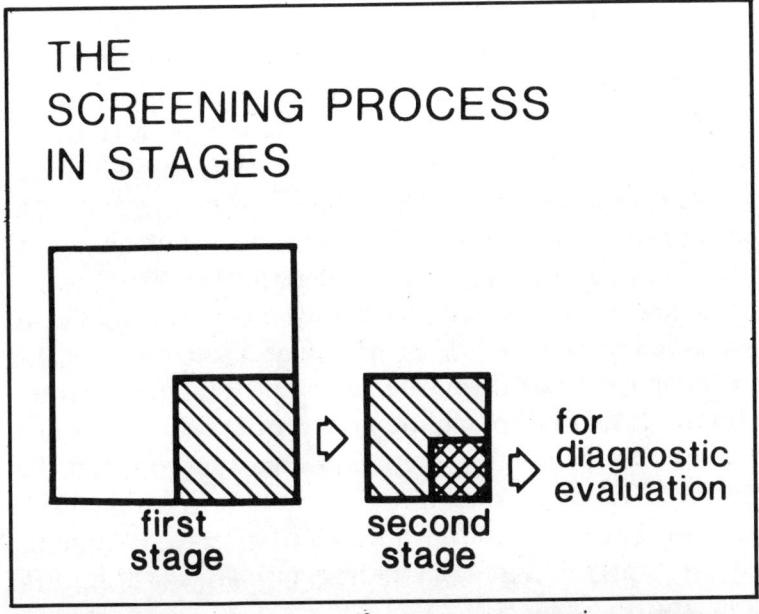

Figure 7. Schematic diagram of a two-stage screening process.

It takes 15 to 20 minutes to administer the DDST to a child and costs about $10. These costs, though moderate, may be too high to permit the routine and periodic screening of large masses of children. We have therefore developed a quicker and more economical prescreen or first screen. Called the Prescreening Developmental Questionnaire (PDQ), this instrument consists of 97 DDST items transformed into questions that can be answered by parents. The questions are arranged in chronological order according to the ages at which 90%

of the children in the original DDST normative sample passed the corresponding DDST item.

From this "master list," an office assistant assigns ten age-appropriate questions for each parent to answer. Children who receive suspect scores are rescreened with the PDQ a week or two later and, if still suspect, referred for a diagnostic evaluation.

A recent study in which 10,000 children were screened showed that the PDQ was the most cost-efficient screening method to use with children whose parents had at least a high school education. Among these higher SES families, 16% required a second PDQ, and the two-stage process identified all the children functioning in the retarded range as determined by independent psychological evaluations.

For screening the children of parents with less than a high school education, however, the PDQ turned out to be less accurate than the DDST. As a result, we developed a short form of the DDST as a more effective prescreen for this lower SES group. The short form identifies as suspect all the children who would be so identified on the full DDST. If one or more of the twelve items on the short form is failed, the full DDST is given. About 25% of the children screened with the short DDST receive suspect scores and need to be given the full test.

SCREENING FOR POTENTIAL SCHOOL PROBLEMS: THE DDST AND HSQ. Until recently, all screening efforts focused on developmental delays. About three years ago, we became interested in a more common problem: school learning problems, particularly among children residing in low socioeconomic environments. Such problems are of major concern, since in these disadvantaged populations the rate of school problems is close to 50%.

We began this part of our research by investigating the predictive accuracy of the DDST in identifying later school problems. Van Doorninck et al. have reported a five-to-six year follow-up study of 151 children who took the DDST between the ages of 3 months and 6

years. At the time of the follow-up, the children were classified as having "school problems" if they met any one of the following criteria:
 (1) achievement test scores below the tenth percentile;
 (2) special education placement or has repeated a grade;
 (3) very severe behavior problems according to teachers' ratings;
 (4) IQ less than 80 on the Stanford-Binet.

The study found that 89% of the children with abnormal DDST scores and 63% of those with scores in the questionable category did have school problems five to six years later. Of the children with normal DDST scores, 62% did not encounter school problems — but 38% did. In other words, a child with an abnormal DDST was very likely to have school problems later, but about a third of the children with normal DDSTs also turned up with later problems. Diagnostic developmental and IQ tests administered early in a child's life also miss a large proportion of children who go on to experience school problems, for various reasons. One is that precursors of school failure may develop at any time in a child's life, after a screening test as well as before.

About four years ago, we began to see limitations in assessing only the child when screening for potential school problems. Emmy Werner has reported that ten times as many children fail in school because of adverse home environments as because of perinatal stress. So we thought it would be worthwhile to look at the child's home environment.

Bettye Caldwell's Inventory of Home Stimulation (STIM) scale seemed appropriate for our purposes, since it had been developed by referring to past studies relating environmental factors to developmental outcomes. We investigated and found a respectable .42 correlation between the STIM used when a child was 12 months old and that child's performance in elementary school. The main drawback of the STIM, which has been rechristened the Home Observation for Measurement of the Environment (HOME), was that it required up to two hours to make a home visit and interview the family.

With the assistance of Dr. Caldwell, we therefore developed the Home Screening Questionnaire (HSQ), to be answered by parents. The questionnaire is written at a fifth-grade reading level and takes about 15 minutes to complete. There are two forms, corresponding to the age groups covered by the HOME scale: birth to 3 and 3 to 6.

Thus far, the HSQ and DDST have been administered to some 1,365 children, and follow-up HOME interviews have been administered to 790 families. It will be several years before we can relate the scores from these assessments to the children's performance at school. In the meantime, as a preliminary estimate of test validity, we have examined the scores in relation to the school records of 191 siblings of the screened children.

Our results show high agreement between the HSQ and HOME scales in identifying sibling school problems. In addition, whereas the DDST identified only about 20% of sibling problems, the HSQ and HOME inventory identified about 70%. This discrepancy is not surprising, since the HSQ and HOME assess an environment that siblings presumably share whereas the DDST score primarily reflects each child's own biological integrity.

School follow-up on the actual children screened in our study will allow us to complete our evaluation. For now, we are optimistic about the usefulness of a combined developmental-environmental assessment in identifying children who are at risk for later school problems.

Bax: Are you worried at all about the accuracy of the parental reports you get on your questionnaires?

Frankenburg: Not really. In my clinical experience over the years, when I've done a lot of Gesell tests with children and also asked mothers whether the children could do something, I had a very high agreement rate between what they told me and what I observed. The trick is to ask questions about things parents could have observed, and also to phrase them in a way that's not leading.

Bax: Were the parents of children with abnormal scores as accurate as the others? In my experience you get a more accurate report from the mother of a child who doesn't have a developmental disorder than from the mother of a child who does, because the parent is often anxious about the disorder.

Frankenburg: When we devised the Prescreening Developmental Questionnaire (PDQ), we found we got good agreement between mothers and outside observers, who would listen to what the mothers said the child could do and then check it, by asking the child to ride a tricycle or whatever. We didn't find any difference in accuracy based on the child's score. We did find a social-class difference: more educated parents tended to underrate the development of their children, and parents with less than a high school diploma tended to overrate it. As a result, we missed some children in the poverty sample and we didn't miss them in the educated sample. That's why we recommend using the short DDST instead of the PDQ with poverty populations.

Lester: You said the DDST isn't racially biased, but couldn't it be accused of bias against lower socioeconomic groups, since they get lower scores? This is a problem with many tests, so I'm wondering what you think of the idea of using local norms in developing test questions. If you're screening poverty or Head Start children, some people would say you should standardize the test on that population.

Frankenburg: We think that's really doing a disservice to the people involved. Essentially, what we're trying to do is identify children who are destined to fail in school. If we were to standardize the test on poverty children, we'd be lowering our expectations for them — and the same high percentage would still fail at school. In our view, what we should do instead of criticizing tests like the Stanford-Binet is take a hard look at society and its injustices.

McCall: Overall, what percentage of the children you screen get abnormal DDST scores?

Frankenburg: Roughly, abnormals and questionables together are 10% — abnormals are 3% and questionables another 7%. These figures are consistent in our own studies and other people's.

McCall: Did you say that using the DDST as well as the HOME scale to predict siblings' school problems didn't work any better than using the HOME scale alone?

Frankenburg: That's right. In a population with a 50% school failure rate, the DDST is going to miss a lot of people, even if it identifies more than the usual 10% as suspect. We were glad to find that the DDST and the HOME had different predictive powers, because otherwise we'd have had to question whether it was worthwhile to use both.

Barnard: We have some data that certainly supports the HOME scale as a good measure during early life. We've collected a great deal of information about environmental, child, and parent variables, and HOME shows the best correlation with later development of any measure we've used. Which items on the HOME scale did you find predicted later school performance?

Frankenburg: Some were items you'd never think of, like whether there were plants in the home, or pets. And whether they tried recipes from the newspaper. Our thought was that perhaps what these items have in common is maternal depression. If a mother is depressed, maybe she doesn't try out recipes or take care of a plant or a dog — and maybe she's not at her best with the baby, either.

Barnard: I'd like to mention a within-class difference that we've found in high-education families. In these families, the items that distinguish children who do well from children who do less well seem to center on the issue of restrictiveness. In lower socioeconomic groups, the issue with correspondingly good predictive power seems to be responsiveness.

Frankenburg: In trying to figure out why poverty infants up to 20 months of age show more advanced development on the DDST than middle-class infants do, we've thought it might be because the poverty infants are less restricted. At older ages, though, a lack of restrictiveness may begin to slide over toward neglect. The adults don't fence the children in, but they don't interact much with them, either.

Bax: Suppose you do succeed in identifying the 50% of poverty children who will probably have school problems. What then?

Frankenburg: That's a good question. At this point I'll just say that the purpose of screening is to facilitate diagnosis at an early stage in the disease or handicapping process. The idea is that through early identification you can modify the morbidity and improve the picture down the road. So it doesn't make much sense to screen for a nonserious condition that can't be treated effectively anyway, like flat feet. Neither does it make sense to expend resources on screening for potential school problems if you're not going to use early identification to try to modify outcome.

Predicting Developmental Outcome: Resumé and Redirection
by Robert B. McCall, Ph.D.

After reviewing several decades' worth of prediction literature, Robert McCall reports some bad news and some good. The bad news is that standardized infant tests administered to children under the age of 2 do not predict later IQ with much accuracy. Both for normal infants and for infants at risk, the best single predictor of developmental outcome is not early test performance but parental education or family socioeconomic status. A low score, McCall suggests, should be regarded chiefly as an indication of current difficulties. The good news is that poor-scoring infants often recover with development, indicating substantial potential for treatment and intervention.

Nearly five decades of research have been devoted to predicting later developmental outcome from standardized assessments made during infancy. This vast literature funnels to a single conclusion: For unselected samples of essentially normal children, individual differences in later developmental status, particularly in intelligence, are not related to any useful extent to individual differences on standardized infant tests administered prior to the age of two.

Despite this conclusion, which has been replicated repeatedly, interest in prediction has been resurrected in the last few years, with a slight change in focus. Now the question is, Can we predict from early infancy those children who will turn out to have defects, abnormalities, or subnormal intelligence in childhood and adulthood?

This renewed interest stems from at least two recent developments. First, the Early and Periodic Screening, Detection, and Treatment program (EPSDT), revised and expanded as the Child Health Assessment Program (CHAP), has meant that hundreds of thousands of youngsters are being screened across the country each year for potential health and developmental disabilities.* Such screening for many physical ailments is precise and accurate. But this is not the case for the early

*Despite the fact that it is the principal screening test for infants and young children in the EPSDT battery and the only infant test mentioned in several major pediatric textbooks, the Denver Developmental Screening Test (discussed by Frankenburg at this conference) is not considered in this paper. The reason is that

prediction of developmental retardation, and accuracy levels seem to be even worse for the detection of social-emotional problems.

A second reason for renewed interest in early prediction of developmental deficit is the increased ability of physicians to salvage infants suffering perinatal traumas and insults. Some of these survivors are at increased risk for adverse CNS conditions later in life. Predicting which high-risk infants will suffer later defects would presumably allow earlier intervention and more opportunities for beneficial treatment.

HOW ACCURATE ARE EARLY PREDICTIONS OF IQ? Most prediction studies have used tests given before the age of three years to predict later IQ. In order to achieve slightly greater comparability, I have restricted the studies surveyed to those reporting results in terms of correlation coefficients. The accuracy of prediction in these studies varies with the nature of the sample, depending on whether it is composed of normal, at-risk, or specifically handicapped infants and children.

In studies of unselected or "normal" individuals, correlations are quite modest from any assessment made prior to age 2 and are not high enough to be clinically useful until childhood, as shown in Table 2. Predictive correlations are slightly higher for samples of infants born at risk for later abnormality (Table 3), but not high enough to make the infant test a clinically useful tool for prediction when used alone. For these omnibus at-risk samples, the pattern of correlations is roughly similar to that of normal samples, though correlations tend to rise at somewhat earlier ages for at-risk groups.

In samples of children with known specific abnormalities or syndromes, are correlations any higher? As shown in Table 4, correlations can be very high for some syndromes at some ages but modest for others. One

very little predictive validity information on the DDST is available, and the research that has been done evaluates categorical predictions to categorical criteria rather than calculating correlations. While ample justification exists for such procedures, the data are not comparable to those presented in the tables here.

Table 2. Correlations Between Infant Test Scores and Childhood IQ for Unselected ("Normal") Samples*

Age of childhood test (years)	Age of infant test (months)				
	1-6	7-12	13-18	19-30	
8-18	.06 (6/4)	.25 (3/3)	.32 (4/3)	.49 (34/6)	.28†
5-7	.09 (6/4)	.20 (5/4)	.34 (5/4)	.39 (13/5)	.25
3-4	.21 (16/11)	.32 (14/12)	.50 (9/7)	.59 (15/6)	.40
	.12†	.26	.39	.49	

Data taken from Anderson 1939; Bayley 1933; Bayley 1954; Birns and Golden 1972; Cattell 1940; Cavanaugh et al. 1957; Elardo et al. 1975; Escalona and Moriarty 1961; Fillmore 1936; Goffeney et al. 1971; Hindley 1965; Honzik et al. 1948; Ireton et al. 1970; Kangas et al. 1966; Klackenberg-Larsson and Stensson 1968; McCall et al. 1972; Moore 1967; Nelson and Richards 1939; Werner et al. 1968.

*Decimal entries indicate median correlation.

†Marginal values indicate the average of the *r's* presented in that row/column.

Reprinted with permission from R. B. McCall, The development of intellectual functioning in infancy and the prediction of later IQ. In J. D. Osofsky (Ed.), *Handbook of Infant Development.* New York: Wiley, 1979

might expect that within a group of infants handicapped in the same way and to approximately the same extent (such as a group with Down's syndrome), correlations would be low because of the restricted range of values. In contrast, for a syndrome that handicaps children in widely varying degrees (such as "mental retardation" or cerebral palsy), variability and stability might be quite great. The data are too skimpy at this point to test this hypothesis.

In my view, there are two major reasons why our attempts at predictions based on infant test scores have not been more successful. One reason is statistical; the other concerns the nature of early development.

STATISTICAL REASONS FOR PREDICTION FAILURES. There are many more infants born at risk than there are children or adults with deficiencies. From the standpoint of human suffering, this is a blessing; from the standpoint of forecasting later development, it is a nightmare.

Table 3. Correlations Between Infant Test Scores and Childhood IQ for At-Risk Samples

Age of childhood test (years)	Age of infant test (months)				
	1-6	7-12	13-18	19-36	
8-18				.71[f] .46[f*] .52[f*]	.56†
5-7	.54[a]	.57[a]			.56
3-4		.37[b*] −.11[b] .48[c]		.86[b]	.40
2	.29[e] .42[d]	.44[b*] .30[b] .07[d] .39[d] .48[e]	.63[d]		.36
	.42†	.31	.63	.64	

The correlations presented above are from [a]Drillien 1961; [b]Hunt 1979; [c]Knobloch and Pasamanick 1960, [d]Siegal et al., 1979; [e]Sigman, Note 1; [f]Werner et al. 1968.

*Sample restricted to subjects scoring below a cut-off at both ages.

†Marginal values are the average of the r's presented in that row/column.

Table 4. Correlations Between Infant Test Scores and Childhood IQ for Clinic and Handicapped Samples

Age of childhood test (years)	Age of infant test (months)			
	1-6	7-12	13-18	19-24
8-18				
5-7	.26[a]	.51[a] .11[d] .73[d] .50[d]		.81[a] .59[d] .76[d] .64[d]
3-4	.20[b]	.64[b]	.72[b] .63[f]	.83[b]
2	.63[a] .36[c]	.76[e] .72[f] .39[g]	.77[e]	

The correlations presented above are from [a]Fishman and Palkes, 1974, spina bifida; [b]Carr 1975, Down's syndrome; [c]Dicks-Mireaux 1966, Down's syndrome, *our calculation*; [d]Fishler, Graliker and Koch, 1964-65, cerebral palsy, congenital anomalies, Down's syndrome; [e]Goodman and Cameron 1978, clinic population; [f]Erickson 1968, "young M.R." [g]Share, Webb and Koch 1961-62, Down's syndrome.

Tables 3 & 4 are reprinted with permission from C. B. Kopp and R. B. McCall, Stability and instability in mental performance among normal, at-risk, and handicapped infants and children. In P. B. Baltes and O. G. Brim, Jr. (Eds.), *Life-Span Development and Behavior*, Vol. 2, New York: Academic Press, in press.

One result of the fact that many at-risk children develop normally is that retrospective studies make risk factors look considerably more important than do prospective studies. That is, among children having one or another defect, the likelihood that a given risk sign was present during infancy may be quite high — several times greater than within a normal population. But even so, infants having the risk sign may be only slightly more likely to develop the defect than those lacking the sign.

For example, in a study of newborn anoxia, Broman found that children who scored in the retarded range at 8 months, 4 years, and 7 years were five to twenty times more likely to have had one or another sign of anoxia at birth than were children who scored in the superior range at those ages. These retrospective data seem to mean that anoxia is a very significant risk sign for retarded development. But when the same sample is viewed prospectively, the conclusion is different. When children with and without signs of anoxia at birth were compared on IQ tests administered during early childhood, the difference between the groups was only about four IQ points. Obviously, many infants who suffered anoxia did not display later deficits.

Moreover, the magnitude of the difference seemed to depend more on sex, race, and socioeconomic class than on the presence or absence of anoxia. Most of the literature I have read indicates that the single best predictor of outcome for high-risk infants (as for unselected groups) is the socioeconomic status of the infant's parents.

In any event, most infants who score poorly on infant tests during the first few months of life, or who are designated at risk because of perinatal complications, recover or eventually develop within the normal range. This means that infant tests have rather high false positive rates. That is, they predict that too many infants will develop subnormally. High false positive rates explain why screening devices are typically used in combination with other diagnostic techniques that help eliminate normals and confirm suspected abnormals.

THE NATURE OF EARLY DEVELOPMENT. A second reason for our difficulties in predicting later abnormality is the nature of early development. I believe there are two characteristics of early development that make it a poor platform from which to predict later status.

The first characteristic is canalization, which means that the members of a species tend to follow a common developmental path, assuming that they remain in environments typical for the species. In the first two years of life, human development is highly canalized. Those who stray from the usual path for one reason or another tend to return promptly when the deflecting circumstance is alleviated. Thus, infants born at risk or with depressed development in the early months show a strong self-righting tendency, especially if they are reared in advantageous environments. As a result, individual differences in the first two years of life are not very predictive and not diagnostically precise.

The second aspect of development that makes prediction difficult is that intelligence is not like a balloon that simply grows bigger as the breath of experience and maturation blows it up. The development of intelligence, and perhaps development in other behavioral domains, proceeds according to a sequence of stages. What determines performance in one stage may be qualitatively different from what determines it in another. This is at the roots of Piaget's conception of cognitive development.

Many psychologists have accepted Piaget's stage theory of cognitive development without considering its implications for the prediction enterprise. Yet a stage theory of development seems to make low predictive correlations almost inevitable. According to my analysis, correlations are in fact somewhat lower when the time period spans a hypothesized stage boundary than for an equivalent period that does not cross a stage boundary. That is, the accuracy of predictions appears to be reduced because of qualitative changes in the nature of mental behavior at different ages. Predictions of abnormalities are also difficult because some disabilities are not manifest until later stages are reached (e.g., language).

ARE INFANT TESTS REALLY WORTHLESS? It would be easy to conclude from my review that infant tests are worthless and should be discarded. I do not subscribe to this view. A low score on an infant test is a risk sign, in the same way — and perhaps with the same level of accuracy — as a history of hypoxia. Both have some significance, even though their predictive power in the absence of other symptoms is modest. If development is indeed highly canalized and proceeds through a sequence of qualitatively different stages, it may be too much to hope that we will be able to forecast the presence of an abnormality before its symptoms are manifest, but this does not rule out nonpredictive purposes for the infant test.

The infant test does, after all, reflect current status. Birth weight is not very predictive of later weight or later health, but it is a decent general sign of current status. We do not ignore weight because it doesn't predict; neither should we ignore the infant test. In addition, when the tests are given periodically they chart relative developmental progress. They may reveal recovery from a depressed beginning, or they could be an important diagnostic sign if relative performance begins to fall consistently after a period of stable scores.

Superseding the prediction issue is the fact that the parents' education or socioeconomic status is the best single predictor of outcome for normals and risk infants alike. While this is bad news for those among us who would like to predict abnormality with infant tests or on medical grounds, it is good news for those among us who want to intervene and help the infants most likely to have developmental difficulties. In addition, newer data (such as that presented by Barnard and Horowitz, this conference) suggest that certain styles of interaction between mother and infant that vary *within* SES groups are related to outcome. Consequently, there is reason to be hopeful about effective parenting and intervention programs.

THE CLINICAL TASK. Some babies go home from the hospital apparently normal but are brought to medical attention later by their parents, who think "something is wrong." Some specialists in high-risk infants are very sensitive to parental concerns and have remarked to me, "If a mother is worried, I listen to her, because most of the time she is correct." In my very limited experience, such pediatric specialists often feel that a low test score has considerably more predictive validity than suggested by the data reviewed here. One reason for this may be that a good pediatrician is a better diagnostician than the infant test. I hope this is the case.

Many other pediatricians, in contrast, respond to a concerned parent and a low test score with the age-old reassurance that "each child is different, one should not compare one child with another, and he'll likely grow out of it." The data reviewed here imply that they will be correct more often than not.

But not always. Some babies showing risk signs will indeed develop a problem. The task is to determine for whom the bell tolls, and the difficulties of doing this in the early months are frustrating to parent and pediatrician alike. The parent senses that something is wrong and desperately wants a firm diagnosis. The pediatrician is reluctant to speak too soon. Both parent and physician are justified in their attitudes, but they often do not understand each other.

On the one hand, the pediatrician needs to display some concern for the parent's anxieties. The situation for the parent may be made worse if the pediatrician dismisses the parent's concerns out of hand. Parents can be told how unusual the atypical behavior is and how likely it is to be a sign of abnormality, and they can be invited to call if the child exhibits other behaviors that worry them. On the other hand, parents need to understand that some defects cannot be diagnosed at an early age even when an unusual symptom is present.

In the meantime, the researchers among us might get

busy reevaluating our screening, detection, and diagnostic procedures and creating much-needed improvements in them.

Carey: I agree with most of what you've said, Bob, but you don't mention two problems I've seen in child development research that lead us to underestimate whatever stability or continuity there is. The first problem is that measurements at two different times often do not assess the same variable. I remember a study I saw a while back saying there is no stability in infant temperament because motor activity is not the same at different ages. But in this study the measure of motor activity for the younger children (one-year-olds, I think) was the number of squares on the floor a child would go across in one minute. At the later age, which I think was 2 years, the measure of motor activity was how many times the child would crank a handle on a box. Well, these behaviors probably don't correlate even when they're measured at the *same* time! How can one say that a lack of correlation shows there is no stability in motor activity?

The other thing that bothers me is that the samples of behavior used in developmental studies are often meager. I've seen studies in which a baby is observed for as little as 20 seconds, which is not a very big chunk of behavior, and much is made of that. I don't think we should expect these little bits of behavior to correlate over time.

McCall: You have certainly identified some fundamental problems with research in developmental science. The issue is whether the problems you mention qualify or negate the general thrust of the data I have presented. Considering your second point first, infant test items tap a variety of behaviors, both mental and motor. Scores on one infant test correlate highly with scores on other infant tests, and attempts to create new tests often result in a return to the old items as a decent sample of such behavior. A major exception is tests based upon Piaget's notions of mental development, and, in general, scores on these tests are less stable and less predictive than scores on traditional tests. So, while the infant tests certainly have their limits, I do not think they assess an isolated, atypical set of behaviors.

Your first point is certainly true — the qualitative nature of mentality is not the same in infancy as in childhood or adulthood — and I fully agree that this fact contributes to poor prediction. But this circumstance is a fact of life and development. It would be nice to have a measure of intelligence that was assessed in the same way at every age (such as the speed of evoked cortical responses to stimulus changes), but I haven't seen it yet. So far, although their nature changes with development, the infant and IQ tests have considerable contemporary validity and utility, and stability of mental test scores is probably higher than for any other behavioral trait yet measured. So from a practical standpoint, I think we are doing as well as we now know how in this regard. I join you in hoping for better things in the future, but I also feel we need to be prepared for the fact that lack of prediction is an accurate reflection of nature.

Frankenburg: You know, Bob, I think some people may misinterpret what you're saying about low predictability. Isn't it true that your conclusions about infant tests are based largely on studies of normal children, such as Nancy Bayley's work and the Fels Institute longitudinal study? As clinicians, many of us see children with marked deviations, and their tendency to "self-right" or to outgrow these things is really quite limited. Take Down's syndrome: would you say that we cannot predict that a child with Down's syndrome is going to have problems later in life?

McCall: No, I wouldn't. I concentrated on cases where

obvious syndromes such as Down's were not present, because it seemed to me that the purpose of screening and of infant tests as a diagnostic tool is less one of confirming a diagnosis of Down's syndrome than of predicting normality or abnormality when manifest symptoms are not present. I did review the literature for predictions within high-risk samples, and I reported on those.

Bax: Still, if a baby scores really low on a developmental assessment at one year, I think his chances of being mentally subnormal later are pretty high.

McCall: Now, I didn't say the likelihood doesn't increase with a low score. But the way I read the literature, a great number of low-scoring babies develop normally. A low score does have more predictive significance than an average score or even a very high one, but I am asking whether the likelihood increases enough to make that score alone clinically useful. I don't think so, at least not in screening populations. But, if you are a pediatrician specializing in high-risk infants who are referred to you, the test may be much more accurate because the base rate of problems in the group you see is much higher — your sample is selected in this regard. I think this fact explains why many pediatricians who specialize in high-risk infants feel the test is useful, more useful than the data seem to indicate. For them it may be.

Brazelton: We haven't mentioned something that I think is the crux of our medical problem, and that is that we look at everything with a pathological model in mind instead of looking for optimality or invincibility or strengths. Adaptability — as indicated by variability and change — may be our best predictor of a good outcome, and invariability or fixation may be evidence of deviance. To me, this is a fascinating implication of the work Frank Duffy has described.

Frankenburg: I've suggested we ought to think not only about child status but about the environment, particularly the home environment.

McCall: I heartily agree with that.

Barnard: It seems to me what you're saying is that we should not use the infant test alone to reach a decision that a child is going to be abnormal. You're not saying that a low score is meaningless. You're just making the point that we need additional confirming evidence from other sources.

McCall: That's right.

Brazelton: Let me suggest again that a lack of predictability is really due to variability, and that variability — change — is probably the best thing we've got in the human organism. It demonstrates the recuperability that we have available to us, and it suggests that early testing might well be used to mobilize resources for the baby rather than just to make a static prediction.

PART TWO
EARLY INTERVENTION: SOME STRATEGIES

Intervention Programs for Infants with Cerebral Palsy: A Clinician's View

by Lawrence T. Taft, M.D.

Lawrence Taft's eloquent defense of intervention programs draws on years of clinical experience with handicapped infants. Taft begins by acknowledging an unpleasant truth: according to outcome studies, the motor abnormalities of infants with cerebral palsy are not likely to be significantly reduced through intervention. But intervention programs have other benefits that are significant indeed. They include improvements in the parents' ability to adapt to their infant's handicap, a better relationship between parents and child, and heightened motivation and self-esteem for the child.

Ongoing informational and counseling sessions for parents are a vital part of a comprehensive intervention program, Taft says. Parents can also be taught to use various postural adjustments to minimize the infant's spasticity and maximize functional competence. Taft's perspective emphasizes the family context of infant development and the need to foster a child's growth as a person, no matter how severe her or his motor impairment.

Is there acceptable research evidence that early intervention changes the natural course of the motor disorder seen in children with cerebral palsy? In my opinion, the answer is no. Is there acceptable research evidence that early intervention minimizes complications or substantially improves motor functioning? I believe not. Like many clinicians, I favor intervention, but my reasons have little to do with the findings of outcome studies.

Outcome research on cerebral palsy is made especially difficult by the unpredictability of the disorder. Some time ago, I had the experience of seeing two infants with similar birth weights, similarly elevated bilirubin levels in the first few days of life, similar signs of possible abnormality on early neurological exams, and similar delays in achieving gross motor landmarks. Yet by the time these infants reached school age, one had developed an incapacitating athetoid cerebral palsy while the other was merely clumsy. I would like to be able to say that the clumsy child had received specific therapeutic intervention and the other child had not, but in fact these were identical twins, raised by their parents without professional help.

I have two reasons for recommending intervention programs even though they apparently do not improve motor outcome significantly. First, animal studies indicate considerable plasticity of brain function. Do the complexities of the human brain make a meaningful reorganization after a cerebral lesion less likely in our species — or more so? If we can discover the right "strings to pull," perhaps secondary pathways can come into play even though a primary circuit remains nonfunctioning. Second, I favor intervention because I am convinced it has broad positive effects not tapped by outcome studies.

BENEFITS OF INTERVENTION. Clinical observation has shown me that intervention programs have the following benefits for motor-handicapped children and their families: (1) better parent-child relationships; (2) child more strongly motivated to try new motor tasks; (3) less parental "shopping"; (4) quicker and less painful adaption by parents to child's handicap; and (5) a happier child.

Some people might consider these results insignificant for, say, a child who still cannot walk independently. I disagree! Growing up without depression, well-motivated and socially competent in spite of a serious handicap, meets my criteria for a positive outcome. So does a result that gives parents a realistic view of the future and helps them feel they have met a difficult challenge as best they could.

At first, many parents react to the news that their infant is handicapped by denying that the handicap is serious or permanent. When this defense against overwhelming grief and anxiety is used, it often leads parents to seek not only a second opinion but a third, fourth, fifth, and sixth. The parents say they want confirmation of the original diagnosis, but of course what they really want is to hear that the diagnosis was wrong. The adverse effect of shopping is not simply the financial drain but the drain on the parents' energy, which may be so great that the child suffers.

Many parents find it impossible just to sit back and accept the consequences of the bad news. When a referral to an early intervention center is given at the time of the diagnosis, at least there is an "upbeat" ending to the interview and not the usual feeling of hopelessness that parents experience. The referral also seems to direct the parents' energy away from seeking other opinions, partly because they are reluctant to postpone the start of therapy.

If the physician offers no specific therapeutic measures at the time of the diagnosis, this intensifies the parents' feeling that all is lost. In desperation, they may seek out therapeutic approaches that are extremely controversial or in the charlatan category.

PARENTAL EDUCATION AND COUNSELING. The more comprehensive intervention programs for children with cerebral palsy include ongoing individual or group sessions for parents. During these sessions, the causes and clinical course of cerebral palsy are discussed and the available medical and surgical therapies reviewed. When parents are helped to try to understand the causes of cerebral palsy, they feel less responsible for their infant's disability. Information on the changing picture seen in many children with cerebral palsy minimizes the parents' anxiety when changes occur. Frank discussion of the controversies surrounding different therapies is also in order, to prepare parents for conflicting advice from well-meaning friends and relatives on such matters as prosthetics and surgery and to equip them for making well-informed decisions of their own.

Parents also need to be told that their child will probably move through the same sequences of functioning as the average child, but at a slower rate. If parents let the child's chronological age determine their expectations and behavior toward the child, they are likely to become increasingly disappointed, and their concern may establish a pattern of failure for the child. It is important that they know the infant's limitations, so that they can play with her or him at an appropriate level and have realistic expectations of progress.

There are many advantages to making the parents active participants in therapy with their child. However, there are also some dangers. The life of the family should not revolve only around the handicapped child; the therapy that parents administer should not consume all their time and energy; and the parents should not relate to the child solely through the therapy. These issues must be discussed with parents, and home visits should be made to assess the family situation.

Supportive counseling is more acceptable to parents when it is part of a larger program and not the sole recommendation made after a diagnosis. Parents find it very difficult simply to talk about a problem. Many say frankly, "Treat our child, not us." Participation in counseling is usually enhanced if the counseling is associated with a program of hands-on therapy for the infant.

For the child who is trying to develop satisfying independent functioning, the help of speech, occupational, and physical therapists can be invaluable. The mode of therapy most often prescribed is the neuro-developmental approach developed by the Bobaths. Although this approach to treatment of movement disorders in infants and children has not been conclusively shown to improve motor outcome, it has other valuable spinoffs for patients and parents.

POSTURAL ADJUSTMENTS. Many spastic infants tend to assume an extensor posture (back arched). This activates the symmetrical tonic neck reflex and results in extension of the arms, which makes voluntary control of

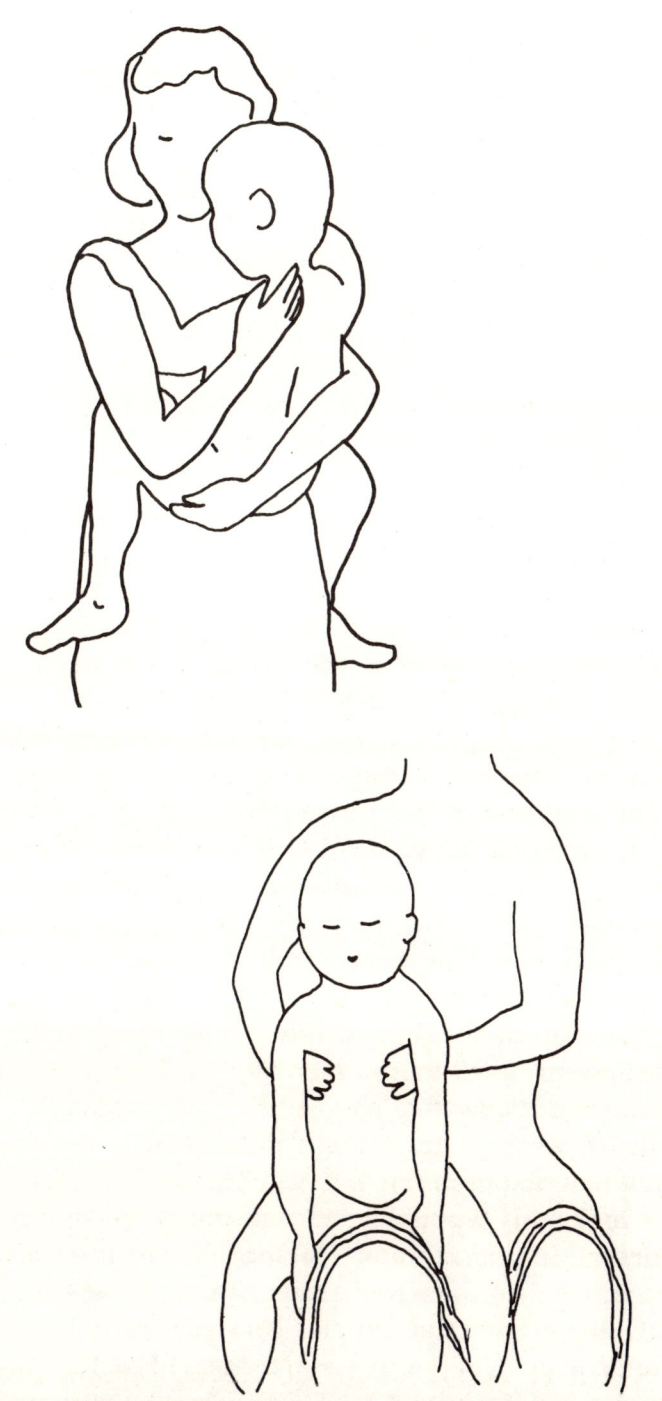

Figure 8. To prevent adduction of the hips in an infant with cerebral palsy, the child's legs should be straddled when the infant is carried or held on the parent's lap.

the arms and hands difficult or impossible. On seeing this, the Bobath therapist will show the parents that placing the infant supine in a sling seat like that of an umbrella stroller helps maintain flexion of the neck and trunk. The slightly rounded position gives the baby better control over the arms and hands and allows him or her to satisfy some needs independently, for example, by sucking a thumb.

I once saw on videotape a powerful demonstration of the negative impact that an abnormal infant's "natural" behavior can have on parent-child relations. The tape showed the first encounter between a mother and baby, which took place when the infant was about 18 hours old. The delivery had been complicated, and the child had an Apgar score of only 5 at one minute and 8 at five minutes. A few hours after birth, the child was examined by a pediatrician and thought to be normal.

The nurse gave the swaddled baby to the mother and left the room. The mother immediately unwrapped the baby. Looking pleased with what she saw, she laid the infant against her arm in order to begin breastfeeding. When placed in the supine position, the infant went into slight extension of the trunk (probably a sign of cerebral irritability). The mother touched the baby's cheek, using the rooting reflex properly. But when the infant's head turned toward the nipple, this activated a definitely abnormal asymmetrical tonic neck reflex. The baby's arm on the chin side went into extension, as if he were "straight-arming" the mother. By now the mother was exasperated and the child, still hungry, was crying, which intensified the primitive reflexes.

What happened next was quite dramatic. The mother finally was able to get the nipple into the baby's mouth, but the infant's sucking movements were uncoordinated. An extensor thrust of the tongue made him seem to spit out the nipple. Now definitely upset, the mother rang for the nurse and handed her the infant, saying, "There's something wrong with the baby."

Unfortunately, the nurse made no inquiries as to what the problem was. If she had, a referral could have been made to a therapist experienced with brain-injured infants. The therapist could have shown the mother how to position the baby in a flexor posture and how to maintain the head in the midline and in flexion. This posture often improves the sucking mechanisms dramatically and makes feedings a rewarding experience for both parties.

I pride myself on being a cautious, conservative, scientific clinician. Yet I constantly must use my clinical judgment when incontrovertible evidence is lacking. My clinical judgment tells me that there is good in early intervention programs, and that to discourage their use is not to the advantage of handicapped children and their families.

McCall: In his introductory remarks, Berry mentioned a statistic to the effect that pediatricians are slow to refer infants to cerebral palsy centers. Do you think they hesitate because they know the centers have no medical cures to dispense?

Taft: That's possible. Another reason may be that the symptoms of cerebral palsy in early infancy can be changeable and hard to read. Take a baby whose central nervous system has been damaged by high bilirubin levels soon after birth. At first, this infant will have a rigid posture and exaggerated reflexes, but over the next few months muscle tone will diminish to normal and beyond. At 10 months, the baby presents as a "floppy" infant with immature motor responses — a raking grasp instead of a thumb-and-forefinger pincer movement. There are no involuntary movements at this age, and an incorrect diagnosis of mental retardation is sometimes made. Over the next 6 months to a year, the infant becomes hypertonic again, and the slow writhing seen in athetosis begins.

Barnard: I think one reason physicians sometimes resist referring children to intervention programs is that medical people tend to look only at child change, generally on standard neurological and developmental measures. The major federal funding agencies do the same thing. For instance, the Bureau of Education for the Handicapped evaluates intervention programs *only* in terms of child change. Intervention programs aren't likely to get high priority when judged in these terms, since the evidence doesn't show much child change. As Larry says, though, we need to consider other things, such as parent behavior and feelings, too.

Brazelton: But it seems to me that the child *does* change with intervention — and also that functional motor outcome improves. Larry has given us several examples of that. The problem as I see it is that we have trouble thinking in functional terms. We're still dominated by the old either/or neurological model.

Parmelee: Larry, don't you find that physical therapists are very much oriented toward trying to improve movement? In programs for children with cerebral palsy, this may be the wrong emphasis.

Taft: This is especially true if the physical therapist is the sole person intervening. The parents and child tend to feel that everything is riding on improvement in motor function.

Parmelee: In our program we have a teacher serve as the child's therapist, because teachers are trained in a more global child-development approach and can learn the specific techniques as they go. Their main goals for the child are normal play and normal self-esteem. The posturing, which they learn from the physical therapist, then becomes a way of allowing for more normal play, and normal play allows for higher self-esteem — we hope.

Taft: In our educational process with parents, we stress the same thing. We explain that we can't predict when a child is going to walk or how good his or her motor functioning is going to be. While growing up, the infant needs chances to experience success and develop self-esteem.

Parmelee: A solid sense of worth is very important for children. If the physical training they receive implies to them that they are going to walk or not be handicapped, they may go into a severe depression as they get older and see that this actually is not the case. The point is not to encourage optimism about the recovery of motor function but to make sure they keep their self-esteem with the handicap.

Duffy: Some children, especially slightly older ones, learn to use their abnormal reflexes to help them do things. For example, a child whose arms seem hopelessly flexed may learn to throw his head and body backwards, so that his arms begin to extend. Then the child can continue the motion. Or a child with a fixed grasp response may find that rubbing the back of the hand on a table triggers momentary extension of the fingers, and use that. Some physical therapists discourage this kind of thing and end up making the child functionally worse.

Brazelton: This is why I question the usefulness of the traditional, neurologically oriented evaluation. If we took a functional approach rather than a fixed approach to the child's problems and progress, we might come up with both better outcomes and better outcome studies.

Taft: I recall a similar example in a boy with athetoid cerebral palsy. This boy still had a primitive tonic neck reflex, so that every time he turned his head to the side, his arm would extend. One of the treatments if you use a doctrinaire approach would be to inhibit that reflex, but what this boy did was make the reflex work for him when he wanted to open a door. If he faced straight toward the door, he couldn't get his hand out to grasp the knob. So he would turn his head to the side. Then his arm straightened out and he could open the door beautifully. There may be many other adjustments that he makes which we know nothing about.

Duffy: If functional competence is the goal, then whether a movement is an abnormal reflex or not isn't the real issue. The issue is whether or not the movement can be incorporated in a sequence when it's wished for.

Early Intervention for Preterm Infants
by Arthur H. Parmelee, Jr., M.D.

Arthur Parmelee's paper poses the question, Why focus only on biological risk factors such as newborn hypoxia when social risk factors such as low socioeconomic status lead to developmental deficits in so many more children? Since 1971, Parmelee and his colleagues have been conducting a major longitudinal study of preterm infants. Its findings have led Parmelee to broaden his conception of risk, and to formulate a correspondingly broad intervention strategy.

An important goal of intervention, Parmelee emphasizes, should be to improve the quality of mother-infant interaction. Often, the best way to help the child is to help the mother. This can be done by interpreting the infant's behavior for her, by showing her how to handle the baby and praising her successful efforts, and by seeing to it that she has the social and financial supports she needs to cope with any special problems her child may have.

An infant "at risk" can be defined as any infant who has a high probability of showing a sensory-motor deficit or a mental handicap in childhood. The preterm infant is the prototypical infant at risk, for preterm infants as a group have a greater incidence of all handicaps than the general population. Even with preterm infants, however, there is difficulty predicting outcome. The incidence of later difficulties may be many times greater in preterm than in full-term infants, but the fact remains that the majority of preterm infants do well. An infant in the lowest gestational-age and birth-weight group runs the highest risk; nevertheless, even some of these infants do well.

All existing follow-up studies indicate that social factors have a great influence on the behavioral and developmental outcome for preterm infants, as they do for full-term infants. These factors must be identified and studied if we are to use social interventions effectively to improve outcome for at-risk infants. Of course, catastrophic outcomes such as cerebral palsy, severe retardation, and severe seizure disorders are not going to be greatly altered by modifications in the social environment. Even in these cases, however, intervention can help the family cope with the difficult situation.

In 1971, Marian Sigman, Claire Kopp, Leila Beckwith, and I began a large-scale longitudinal study of preterm infants that is still in progress. We found that we were unable to predict from gestational age, birth weight, or any neonatal event the child's cognitive status on standard measures at 2 or 5 years. By observing the infants' development carefully with multiple assessments throughout the first year, however, we could predict 2-year and 5-year cognitive behavior at modest levels of significance. Of these assessments, those administered toward the end of the first year, particularly the Gesell developmental test, contributed most to the prediction.

SOCIAL INFLUENCES ON DEVELOPMENT. In the first and second year, mother-infant interaction and other social factors played an increasingly large role in the behavioral development of the infant. The language spoken in the home and the socioeconomic status of the family also became increasingly important in determining the cognitive performance of the children with age.

Chronologically, one of the first "environmental factors" in a preterm infant's life that needs to be considered is the emotional problems of the mother. Most early births are unexpected and unprepared for, and there is often agony over the survival and long-term health prospects of the baby. The mother also feels guilt and loss of self-esteem because she has been unable to carry the infant to term. The poor condition of the infant at birth may mean she is denied physical intimacy, making the associated emotional commitment harder to achieve.

Most nurseries try to provide support for the mother while her preterm infant is in the nursery. Physical intimacy with the baby is encouraged by the nurses whenever possible. Nurses, doctors, and social workers try to provide opportunities for the mother and father to discuss their feelings about the crisis of the preterm birth.

In interviewing parents of newborn preterm infants, Minde found that the number of visits to the nursery and amount of interaction with the infant depended on characteristics of the parents' personal lives. The mother who felt unloved by her own mother as a child and who seemed isolated as an adult, receiving little or no support from family and friends during the infant's neonatal period, was the mother least likely to visit and interact with her infant in the nursery. It is important to recognize that many parent behaviors are functions of their personal feelings, past histories, and home environments. Professionals need to be nonjudgmental about parental responses to the intense emotional experience of having a preterm infant, even when the parents' behavior seems inappropriate to the situation.

CONTINUITY OF CARE. In devising some kind of support system for the families of preterm infants, provision for continuity of care when the baby leaves the hospital is essential. We have tried having the nurse or physician who will see the baby later begin getting acquainted with the family in the nursery before discharge. This person should maintain close contact with the family by phone and through visits during the infant's first weeks at home.

Once an infant is settled at home, interactions with the mother or primary caregiver begin to dominate his or her daily life. In general, the behavior of preterm infants is similar to that of full-term infants if the ages are corrected. However, a preterm baby may provide the mother with fewer signals and less responsiveness than most full-term infants would. Although this behavior might be expected to compound the initial bonding problem, in our study we found instead that mothers of the weaker or sicker babies tried to compensate for their infants' deficits by increasing their interactional efforts. We think the supportive medical care provided through the study may have helped make this possible.

If a mother was able to sustain good interaction with the baby at 1 and 8 months, the infant showed enhanced general competence when tested at 9 months and 2 years. We also found that mothers who continued to provide good mother-infant interaction at 2 years had infants who performed better at 5 years on the Stanford-Binet test.

Thus, mother-infant interaction is significant in promoting later development. The variables that determine the frequency and style of the interaction are not entirely known. Characteristics of the infant and the emotional characteristics and personality of the mother seem to be equally important.

Life circumstances such as the ordinal position of the infant also affect the relationship. Mothers in our study were most successful in establishing intense reciprocal relationships with their first-born infants, perhaps because they had more time and energy to interact with these infants.

The primary language of the family influenced the outcome assessments of the children in our group, with the foreign-language group doing less well than the English-speaking group. The effects of language were compounded by socioeconomic status. With poorer mothers, other factors and stresses in their lives frequently had higher priorities than the infant.

HELPING THE MOTHER HELP THE CHILD. Interventions directed toward improving mother-infant interaction have taken various forms. Interpreting the individual infant's behavior to the mother is an important step. It is also helpful to model techniques of dealing with the baby for the mother and to reinforce the mother's successful spontaneous interactions with the child.

Our intervention program was not successful in all cases. In comparing the characteristics of families of successful and unsuccessful cases, the most striking differences were in the social circumstances of the two groups. In the intervention-failure group there were more marital problems and more changes in the infant's caregivers, more siblings, more economic problems. These factors all seemed to contribute to the low priority of the infant in the family. Efforts at comprehensive intervention must therefore go beyond the mother-infant interaction and include an understanding of the mother's coping ability, support services for her mental health, and economic support for the family, including adequate, stable day care for the infant and siblings when the mother must work.

In summary, mothers' interactions with their infants influence the behavioral outcome of all infants including infants at medical risk. The infant's behavioral capacity controls the form of the mother-infant interaction only to some degree. The mother's feelings of competence and her success in helping her infant achieve a favorable outcome depend in great measure on the mother's own emotional history, her expectations of herself with regard to infants with special problems, and the social and financial support she has in carrying out her perceived role. Interventions should, therefore, be broad-based and concerned with these factors as well as with the details of mother-infant interaction at any particular time.

Brazelton: Tell us more about the effects of a family's primary language.

Parmelee: Those were interesting findings, because they relate to our thinking about the links between biological risk and school problems. Ordinarily, it seems, when a child with a school problem is found to have had hypoxia or some other biological difficulty as a newborn, we blame the school problem on the neonatal event. But in our preterm sample, the children from Spanish-speaking families scored some 20 points below average for the sample as a whole on the Binet IQ test at age 5. We recognize that this test is totally inappropriate for assessment of their true intelligence even though given by a Spanish-speaking tester. Nonetheless, the test scores suggest that these children, despite normal intelligence, are likely to have school problems independent of biological risk. When you consider that immigrant groups often produce a disproportionate number of premature infants, because of poor prenatal care, then you can see you get a distorted picture if you try to analyze school problems without thinking of the child's primary language and biological problems as separate risk factors.

Lester: Are you suggesting that we should add the concept of social risk to that of biological risk?

Parmelee: If we wish to predict behavioral outcome, yes. Obstetricians have devised biological measures — the Apgar score is one of them — that do quite well at predicting which infants will die or be very sick at birth. But predicting newborn mortality and predicting later behavioral outcome are two totally different problems.

I'd like to show you a table summarizing data from the large collaborative project on the IQs of more than 8,000 children at age 4. These were term infants. On this table, biological risk is represented by a low Apgar score, and social risk is represented by a mother with no more than an elementary-school education. As you can see, there is an IQ difference of only 4 points between the low-Apgar and high-Apgar groups. But the difference between the highest and lowest maternal-education groups is 30 IQ points. Clearly, the social factor is swamping the biological one. Of course, the biological factor is still there, so we have to deal with that, too.

Table 5. Mean IQ at Age 4, by Apgar Score and Maternal Education, of 8,000 Full-Term White Children

Maternal education (in years)	Child's Apgar score 5 minutes after birth	
	0-6	8-10
6 or less (N = 238)	90.5 (10)	96.9 (228)
7-9 (N = 1,427)	96.6 (59)	99.4 (1,368)
10-12 (N = 5,146)	101.5 (182)	104.9 (4,964)
13 or more (N = 1,233)	119 (29)	114.8 (1,204)
Mean	101.8 (280)	105.2* (7,764)

*$p = < .001$

Adapted from Drage, J.S., Berendes, H.W., and Fisher, P.D. The Apgar scores and four year psychological examination performance. Pan American Health Organization Scientific Publication **185**: 222, 1969.

Bax: Certain types of cerebral damages do persist into later life, and these children have specific problems that are very predictable. If a child in your sample had pathological brain damage, did your assessment techniques pick it up?

Parmelee: Yes, but not in the newborn period. I want to emphasize, though, that our main concern was not neurological damage but success in the classroom and in the social world more broadly. Basically, we wanted to know whether the baby was going to have enough trouble that we needed to put a lot of effort into helping the mother, whether the source of the trouble was an injured brain or something else.

Bax: If you're trying to predict general functioning, then unless the brain damage is fairly gross you're much better off, as you've indicated, to look at other factors and stop worrying about the biological ones.

Taft: On a clinical basis, Hawley, do you think we're ever going to come up with a practical way of assessing risk and intervening in ways that benefit high-risk infants?

Parmelee: I can address that question from the standpoint of the small number of cases of cerebral palsy that occurred in our sample. We were not able to identify these infants in the neonatal period, as I've said. At 4 months, 11 babies performed very poorly on the Gesell exam. Five of these babies soon manifested clear evidence of cerebral palsy. At 6 months there were some symptoms, and at 9 months there was no question. The 6 babies who had done poorly earlier but did not develop cerebral palsy were performing quite well by 9 months.

As a clinical tool, then, a neuro-behavioral assessment at about 9 months should identify most babies with cerebral palsy and other serious neurological problems. For practicing pediatricians, I would strongly recommend a play-observation session in addition to a routine physical. If pediatricians and family practitioners were to become accustomed to making such a neuro-behavioral evaluation of all their 9-month-olds, I think we would become very skillful at identifying deviations in development.

An Ecological Approach to Parent-Child Relations

by Kathryn E. Barnard, R.N., Ph.D.

In "An Ecological Approach to Parent-Child Relations," Kathryn Barnard shows how much can be learned about the context of an infant's life through careful observation of such ordinary activities as sleeping and feeding. Assessments of these behaviors seem to show, for example, that the parents of infants with problems are willing to work extra hard during the baby's first few months to compensate for the child's unresponsiveness and other difficulties. Toward the child's first birthday, however, there is evidence of parental "burnout." If further research indicates that the super-parent/burnout sequence is a common one, it will constitute a strong case for early intervention aimed at improving parent-child relationships.

In my experience with longitudinal studies of infants and their parents over the past 10 years, I've been impressed with the success of most parent-child interaction systems. For instance, the research literature of the Seventies seems to tell us that the parents of premature infants act to compensate for the infants' problems during the early months. They are "super parents." This picture is similar to the one I have developed through clinical work with handicapped children and their families. I found that when parents of a handicapped child knew how to structure the child's environment in ways that promoted learning or reduced behavior problems, they did so far beyond the endurance of parents of normal children. I also learned that my feedback to these parents was very important in maintaining their interest and hope. The handicapped child is often less responsive than the normal child, making feedback from another source more necessary.

In thinking about the ecology of the developing child, one must try to envision a fluid relationship between child variables and parent variables, and between child-parent variables and variables in the larger environment. My colleagues and I have developed some scales for assessing this fluid parent-child-environment system that have proved particularly useful in looking at problems of prematurity. The assessments can be used as a basis for a supportive and therapeutic relationship with parents.

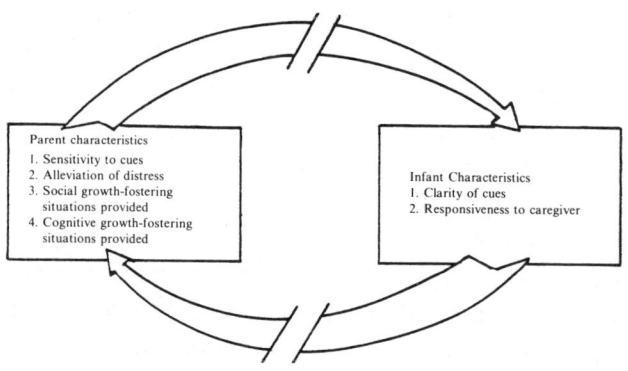

Figure 9. The Barnard model of parent-child interaction.

THE PARENT-CHILD SYSTEM. The interactional model shown in Figure 9 highlights a basic question about the parent-child relationship: Does communication occur? Signals may be given by parent or child, but unless a dyad shares a similar interpretation of those signals, communication will be poor. Important themes that need communicating during the early period of life include need, comfort, safety, trust, attraction, affection, and competence.

The model proposes four communications tasks for the parent and two for the child. Our assessment scales are organized around these tasks. If an infant's cues are difficult to interpret, or if the parent perceives very little positive feedback when trying to interact with the infant, then the parent-infant adaptive process is interrupted and the child's development may suffer. If the parent does not respond to the infant's cues, fails to alleviate distress, or fails to provide growth-fostering situations, the parent-child interaction system can break down, and this too will have a negative influence on the child's development.

In assessing parent-child interaction, we have drawn on Sander's description of four levels of adaptive adjustment between infant and parent during the first year. According to Sander, the central concern of parent and infant during the first few months is the infant's biological rhythms. After about 4 months, issues that are more clearly social begin to take priority.

The assessment instrument we use between birth and 4 months is a sleep-activity record. Called the Nursing Child Assessment Sleep/Activity (NCASA) Record, it resembles the sleep-activity diary used by Gesell and later by Parmelee. It provides a form on which the mother keeps an exact record, hour by hour, of when her baby sleeps and is awake.

We compared the sleep patterns of a population of preterm infants and a population of term infants at 11 weeks of living age. The comparisons, which are detailed in a thesis by Nancy Encke, were based on living age because we feel that it is difficult in a dynamic interaction for a parent to be constantly correcting for gestational age. The parent reacts to the "here-and-now" behavior of the child. We found significant differences between the term and preterm groups on total amount of sleep, with the preterm infants sleeping more. Preterms also slept more during the daytime, had shorter sleep and awake periods and thus more sleep-wake transitions, and showed more night awakenings.

When the children were 2 years old, we were interested to discover a negative correlation for the preterm group between amount of sleep in early infancy and score on the Bayley mental scale at 24 months: Two-year-olds who had slept more during their first few months of life tended to receive lower mental-development scores. This finding has influenced our thinking about the ecological relationship between the preterm infant's sleep-wake behavior and the ongoing caretaking environment.

Sleep variables were also correlated with the mother's feeling of attachment to the infant. Infants with longer sleep periods had mothers who reported taking longer to feel close to their infants.

We propose that the effects of an infant's sleep and activity pattern relate to opportunities for interaction. An infant who is sleeping more is depriving the system by offering relatively few such opportunities. Thus, communication about basic issues — especially need, attraction, affection, and competence, we think — is altered.

After 3 months of age, many of an infant's cues are more social in nature, and it becomes more feasible to observe parent-child interaction in the traditional sense of social communication. We have developed two scales that can be used to record observations of mother-infant pairs during the 3- to 12-month period. The first, called the Nursing Child Assessment Feeding Scale (NCAFS), is for recording observations during feeding sessions. The second, called the Nursing Child Assessment Teaching Scale (NCATS), is for recording parent and child behaviors during a teaching task. Both scales are organized around the four communications tasks of the parent and two of the child that were shown in Figure 9. The observer is asked to rate parent and child on 10 to 15 items under each task.

INFANTS AND PARENTS AT 4 MONTHS. At 4 months of living age, a time when theory emphasizes the importance of social signaling by the child, Anita Spietz, my research colleague, found in both teaching and feeding interactions that the premature infant provided less clear cues and was less responsive to the parent. Further analysis revealed many child items that were passed significantly less frequently by premature infants. In the feeding observations, those items dealt with the child's signaling a readiness to eat, showing a build-up of tension at the beginning of the feeding, moving smoothly and coordinately during the feeding, laughing or smiling during the feeding, actively resisting food being offered, and having few state changes. Prematures also did less vocalizing or smiling in response to the parents' vocalization, and they explored or reached out to parents less often than did term infants.

Prematures failed many more items in the teaching situation at 4 months than they did on the feeding scale. In fact, out of a total of 23 child items, prematures did as well as term infants on only 7. The teaching situation is faster-paced and more novel for the infant than a feeding, and apparently it was more difficult.

At this same time, 4 months, the parents of term and preterm infants differed on only a few items. Overall, our observations at this time led us to believe that problems in interactions between preterm infants and their parents are caused mainly by unclear cues and a lack of responsiveness on the part of the infant.

INFANTS AND PARENTS AT 8 MONTHS. At 8 months, in the feeding situation, the premature infants had become much more similar to term infants in the clarity of their cues, but they still were not as responsive. The mothers of prematures showed less sensitivity to their children's cues than they had at 4 months.

In the teaching situation, preterm and term infants scored similarly on both clarity of cues and responsiveness. The parents of preterm infants were slightly more sensitive to cues than they had been at 4 months, but fewer did well in the social-emotional growth-fostering category. Specifically, there was less parental laughing or smiling at the child during the teaching, and less praise for the child's efforts.

At 8 months, then, the system balance has changed. The preterm infants have become more responsive, generally resembling term infants of the same living age. However, the parents of the preterms — who earlier put out so much effort — now show less sensitivity and emotional responsiveness than they had. This finding suggests a "burnout" phenomenon in parents of children with problems.

SYSTEM DEFICITS. Most studies comparing preterm and term infants conclude that when conceptual age is taken into account, there are few differences between the two groups. The differences that do exist are in the direction of the preterm infants being less socially responsive — smiling less and engaging in less eye contact, for example. Our data confirm these differences.

It is our contention that the system of parent-child interaction during the early months is at a deficit because of the preterm infant's unclear cues and unresponsiveness to the caregiver. At a later age, this deficit takes its toll. The many months of social conditioning that the parents have experienced seem to lead to reduced sensitivity and growth-fostering when the infant is older. Whether this changes at a later time, during the second year, is a question that needs study.

A final comment should be made about the larger environment of parent and child. Of all the mediating variables that we have studied in the past few years, the combination that seems to make the most difference for parent-child interaction includes three items: involvement of the father in the pregnancy as the mother perceives this, amount of life stress the parents are experiencing, and amount of support they feel is available for them in their environment. I think these items show that our attempts to further the recovery of infants or families who have had problems should extend beyond the parent-child dyad itself. The dynamics of that two-person system are inevitably influenced by outside events, for better or for worse.

McCall: Your sleep record is very detailed. Do parents object to filling it out?

Barnard: We've found that actually mothers are very interested in keeping these data. We've used the sleep-activity record many times, not only in the study I've described but in other work, and I think it's a good clinical tool. Besides helping the parents see what's happening with the child, it gives us a piece of clinical information to work with them on.

Carey: I like your conceptualization of the interaction at feeding time. I wonder if you've considered adding some more subjective things such as the degree of satisfaction and fulfillment the mother gets from this activity. That might be rather important.

Barnard: We do ask the mother how she felt about the feeding, and I agree this is important. I remember watching a feeding that lasted for about an hour and a half. The mother went on and on about how much fun it was to feed the baby. We showed her the videotape afterwards because she wanted to see it, and she said, "Boy, I look bored, don't I?" But at discharge this particular mother had a very high degree of confidence in her ability to take care of the baby. She felt really good about herself.

Lester: Did you gather any data on fathers?

Barnard: Yes, though mainly through the mothers' perceptions. We assessed the father's involvement during pregnancy, as I've said. We also asked about father involvement in childcare — how much he helps with diapering, how much time he spends with the child, that sort of thing. This may surprise you, but we found a positive correlation between father involvement in childcare at 4 months and more problems of various sorts later. At several other points in our data, too, problems in the mother-child interaction were accompanied by increased father involvement.

Brazelton: How do you interpret the correlation? You don't want to suggest that a helpful father makes for more problems, do you?

Barnard: We think the increased involvement is telling us something about the stress the family is under. The father seems to be responding to problems in the system — pitching in to help. With infants who have more problems later, we also see a higher assessment by the mother of her psychosocial assets, that is, of the amount of support she's getting from her environment.

Brazelton: So you see father involvement as an index of family stress.

Barnard: Yes. What we're studying now, which may be related, is the drop in the involvement of parents of preterm and handicapped children that takes place by about a year. At first, these parents put a tremendous amount of effort into what might be called the social conditioning of the unresponsive child, but this is followed some months later by what looks like burnout. The possibility that the superparent/burnout sequence is a common one has greatly influenced my thinking about the infant-intervention movement.

Intervention Strategies Using Temperament Data
by William B. Carey, M.D.

Most parents, struck by their children's individuality, find infant temperament an easy concept to accept.

Until recently, however, most scientists seemed to regard the idea with skepticism. In 1963, Thomas, Chess, and Birch reported a ground-breaking study showing that it was possible to place some 60% of babies into one of three temperamental categories. Since that time the notion of intrinsic differences in behavioral style has gained credence in professional and academic circles, though it is still controversial today. In the paper that follows, William Carey discusses clinical interventions based on information about temperament.

This report describes three ways in which data on temperament can aid the clinician in fostering parent-child interaction. First, general educational discussions about temperament between clinician and parent can provide parents with background information that will help them see their child in better perspective. Second, a specific temperament profile of the child can be obtained by using questionnaires such as the ones we have developed. Such a profile gives parents a more organized picture of their child's behavior and sometimes reveals distortions in their perceptions of it. Third, the clinician can attempt to improve parent-child interaction by suggesting helpful changes in parental management.

Before discussing these three levels of intervention, I should briefly review what is now known about children's temperament.

THE STUDY OF TEMPERAMENT. Temperamental differences were recognized at least as early as ancient Greece. Only in the twentieth century have behavioral scientists generally ignored intrinsic behavioral characteristics and overstressed the importance of the environment. Though it is little appreciated in the United States, two of the principal architects of modern environmentalism, Pavlov and Freud, both wrote of intrinsic individual behavioral differences. At present, most behavioral scientists agree that we are in an interactionist period: organismic and environmental factors, working together, are thought to determine behavior and personality.

Over the years, various conceptualizations of temperament have emerged. Today, the most useful definition of temperament is "behavioral style." Temperament is the "how" of behavior in contrast to the "what" (abilities) and the "why" (motivation).

In their longitudinal study of white middle-class New Yorkers in the early years of life, Thomas, Chess, and their coworkers described nine temperamental characteristics: activity, rhythmicity, approach, adaptability, intensity, mood, persistence, distractibility, and sensory threshold. From these nine traits they derived three clinically significant clusters. The *difficult child* is arrhythmic, low in approach and adaptability, intense, and negative. The *easy child* has the opposite profile: rhythmic, approaching, adaptable, mild, and positive. The *slow-to-warm-up child* is like the difficult child in being low in approach and adaptability and negative in mood, but he or she tends to react mildly and is relatively low in activity. About 60% of infants can be categorized by this system. (The others have been designated *intermediate.)*

Note that Thomas and Chess used a white, middle-class sample. Other ethnic and socioeconomic status groups may have different tolerances for some "difficult" traits, as Thomas and Chess themselves have shown with a Puerto Rican sample in New York. Also, the difficulty of these characteristics for caretakers changes somewhat with the age of the child.

Is temperament inherited? Is it stable or does it change? These are complex issues. Temperamental characteristics seem to be partly genetic, but they are also influenced by the prenatal and postnatal environment. The magnitude of the genetic contribution to temperament is hard to ascertain, since even newborn behavior is not exclusively a matter of genes. Furthermore, not all genetically determined characteristics are evident at birth. As for stability and change, there is evidence for both. Temperamental traits *can* change — and yet, often, they do not.

GENERAL EDUCATIONAL DISCUSSIONS. The most superficial level of intervention using data on temperament is educational discussions between the clinician and parent. In talking with parents, the concept of normal individual differences can be presented. It can be discussed in general terms or in relation to instructions about feeding, sleeping, crying, elimination, and so on. The clinician may draw upon background material such as that just reviewed. These discussions can take place at almost any time, from before delivery through adolescence.

By this means parents should get a greater awareness of and respect for normal individual differences in behavior. They can better appreciate that some predispositions are present in children at birth, and that disagreeable behavior in a child is not all traceable to faulty parenting or brain malfunction. For example, a mother may find helpful the knowledge that an infant's slow approach to food or people may be a temperamental characteristic and not a sign of parental inadequacy. Similarly, toddlers who persist at explorations may be demonstrating a normal trait that is a nuisance now but should stand them in good stead when formal learning begins. The highly active preschool child is more likely to be normal than to be overstimulated or to have a malfunctioning brain. Therefore, standard child-rearing advice that works for one child may be inappropriate for another.

Before the advent of refined interview and questionnaire techniques, such general discussions were as far as the clinician could go — and they may be as far as some want to go even now. But one need not stop at this point.

DETERMINING INDIVIDUAL PROFILES. My colleagues and I have developed four questionnaires that can be used to obtain temperament profiles of particular children. Some sample items from the infant and toddler scales are shown in Table 6. Questionnaires for ages 3-7 and 8-12 are also available. Each questionnaire includes about 95 items on which the parent is asked to rate the

Table 6. Sample Items from the Temperament Questionnaires for Infants and Toddlers

From the Infant Temperament Questionnaire (age 4 to 8 months):
1. The infant eats about the same amount of solid food (within 1 oz.) from day to day.
2. The infant is fussy on waking up and going to sleep (frowns, cries).
3. The infant plays with a toy for under a minute and then looks for another toy or activity.
4. The infant sits still while watching TV or other nearby activity.
5. The infant accepts right away any change in place or position of feeding or person giving it.

From the Toddler Temperament Scale (age 1 to 3 years):
1. The child gets sleepy at about the same time each evening (within one-half hour).
2. The child fidgets during quiet activities (story-telling, looking at pictures).
3. The child takes feedings quietly with mild expression of likes and dislikes.
4. The child is pleasant (smiles, laughs) when first arriving in unfamiliar places.
5. The child's initial reaction to seeing the doctor is acceptance.

child's reactions to specific situations from 1, almost never, to 6, almost always. An open-ended request for the parent's impressions of the child appears at the end.

The rating scales on all four temperament questionnaires have high test-retest reliabilities, high internal consistencies, and reasonably high external validity. The general impressions requested on the last page tend to agree with the ratings but are frequently different. Discrepancies between the two are often informative. Questionnaire data should be supplemented by interviewing and observations to get a fuller picture of the interaction.

The more organized, objective view of the child provided by these scales can be valuable in two ways. First, it is useful to identify difficult and slow-to-warm-up children. Most parents of difficult infants do not need to be told that their babies are a challenge, but they are often only dimly aware of the nature of the problem. To know that the difficult characteristics are inborn but usually improve takes a great load of guilt off their shoulders and allows them to respond to their infants with less anger and apprehension. Also, parents often blame themselves unjustly for the timidity seen in the slow-to-warm-up child. However, parents sometimes live fairly harmoniously with these two kinds of children and do not complain about them.

Even without specific advice from the clinician, the process of identifying the child's characteristics may provide the parents with enough insight to make healthy shifts in interaction patterns. An example is the mother who wisely realized that her infant's intensity was just part of a flamboyant style and that she did not need to continue to respond to every yell. This alteration of perspective has been called reframing.

The other principal value in determining the child's specific profile is that major discrepancies between ratings and parental perceptions of temperament may signal problems. This situation is illustrated by the mother who because of her personal problems viewed her boy as more difficult than average, though she rated him as quite easy on the questionnaire items.

In discussing questionnaire results with parents, it is best to avoid the use of labels such as "difficult." When requested, the child's profile can be described in terms of characteristics (rather intense, fairly regular) rather than by means of diagnostic labels, which may be misunderstood. If parents do not ask for the results of a routinely performed temperament profile and if the interaction and development seem normal, I do not feel obliged to discuss the test findings.

INFLUENCING PARENT-CHILD INTERACTION. When there is a developmental or behavioral problem stemming from a temperament-environment interaction, the clinician may be able to influence the interaction favorably and improve the behavioral adjustment by suggesting alternative patterns of parental handling. In addition, parents can be helped to live in a more tolerant and flexible manner with the child's behavioral style, as by providing an active child with more space. Intervention at this level involves supplying both diagnostic insight and advice on what to do.

A difficult temperament may lead to behavior problems, but the two are not the same thing and should not be confused. Temperament is a matter of style, whereas behavioral maladjustment is a chronic disturbance of social relationships or task performance. For example, a volatile temper could be attributed to behavioral style; social isolation because of the temper becomes a behavior problem. Clinical intervention in the interaction should aim to improve the behavioral adjustment of the child, not alter the behavioral style.

Problems of scholastic adjustment are a second area in which the clinician can fruitfully influence the temperament-environment interaction. Several studies have established that scholastic adjustment is affected by temperament. In four independent studies, the characteristic of adaptability, especially, has been shown to be related to teachers' assessments of children's intelligence and adjustment, to neurological referrals, and to scores on academic achievement tests. Recognition of the child's behavioral style often aids in understanding and dealing with these problems.

Teachers are beginning to think more acceptingly about the once unfashionable concept of temperament, but misunderstandings are still evident. Difficult children are often spoken of as immature because of such behavior as temper outbursts and inflexibility. One may question the value of holding a child back for this sort of "immaturity." Slow-to-warm-up children are frequently described as insecure. They may be reluctant to begin new tasks, but once through the initial phases they are just as sure of themselves as their peers.

Perhaps the major misinterpretation at present concerns school children who are low in adaptability and attention span and high in activity. These characteristics tend to cluster together; in fact, the cluster was found in 22% of the children on whom our questionnaire for 3- to

7-year-olds was standardized. These children are apparently the ones being given the label "hyperkinetic" or "minimal brain dysfunction" (and now "attention deficit disorder") by teachers, psychologists, and physicians. However, there is little evidence that these children have anything wrong with their brains, nor do they seem to benefit in any way from being given these rather meaningless labels.

Several additional areas of clinical concern may be related to temperament, but research on them is just beginning. Outstanding among them is the influence of temperament on physical illness — its incidence, manifestations, and management. Temperament-environment conflicts or mismatches may also be related to such diverse problems as child abuse, failure to thrive, and obesity.

SUMMARIZING RECOMMENDATIONS.

(1) Pediatricians, family practitioners, and other clinicians should learn about differences in temperament and actively educate parents about them. Parents gain thereby a background knowledge of individual variations against which to understand their own child. The clinician who wants to review the literature might begin with *Temperament and Development* by Thomas and Chess and my recent chapter in *The Uncommon Child*, edited by Lewis and Rosenblum.

(2) Clinicians should acquaint themselves with the available measurement techniques and consider their routine use. The questionnaires we have developed help sharpen parents' views of their children as individuals. They may also aid the parents in perceiving and interacting with their children in healthier ways.*

*Editor's note. The questionnaires developed by Dr. Carey and his coworkers can be obtained by professional persons by writing to the people listed below. Their authors request a contribution of $5 per scale to cover expenses.

1. Infant Temperament Questionnaire (4 to 8 months) available from Dr. William B. Carey, 319 West Front Street, Media, PA 19063.
2. Toddler Temperament Scale (1 to 3 years) available from Dr. William Fullard, Department of Educational Psychol-

(3) Using both general knowledge about temperament and specific information about a particular child, clinicians should attempt to influence disharmonious interactions when secondary symptoms have arisen or seem likely to. While changing the temperament characteristics (other than perhaps pharmacologically) may be beyond us now, alterations in interaction patterns may bring about better behavioral adjustment.

The nature and extent of the intervention depends on the judgment of the clinician.

Brazelton: When do you administer your first questionnaire?

Carey: I usually send it to the mother in the mail at about 6 months, so that it's available for discussion at the 8-month visit.

Lester: Does the questionnaire really assess the child, do you think, or are you tapping how the mother feels about the child?

Carey: We try to do both. The main body of the questionnaire asks for fairly precise descriptions of the child's behavior. On the last sheet, the mother is requested to give her general impressions or perceptions.

Frankenburg: If you're going to use the scale in telling the mother what she might do differently toward the child, then one might say the only relevant thing is how she perceives the child. Sometimes what you need to do may be to deal with the mother's perceptions.

Carey: Both ratings and perceptions are relevant clinically. However, I'd like to call attention to what

ogy, Temple University, Philadelphia, PA 19122.
3. Behavioral Style Questionnaire (3 to 7 years) available from Dr. Sean C. McDevitt, Devereux Center, 6436 East Sweetwater, Scottsdale, AZ 85254.
4. Middle Childhood Temperament Questionnaire (8 to 12 years) available from Ms. Robin L. Hegvik, 307 North Wayne Avenue, Wayne, PA 19087.

I call the three maternal-perceptions fallacies. The first is to refer to questionnaire ratings of difficult as "maternal perceptions of difficult temperament" without regard for what the mothers' perceptions actually are. Ratings and perceptions can be different. The other two are that temperamental differences are all in the mind of the mother and that mothers are totally unreliable reporters of infant behavior.

Taft: Chess and Thomas studied infants during the first 3 months of life, didn't they? They wanted to get at pure temperamental patterns that might be due to inherited characteristics of the nervous system. But to assess temperament in older infants and children — I don't know how reliable that would be. By that time, the child's behavior has been colored by environmental experiences.

Carey: Temperament is not entirely inborn. It's how the child behaves at any given point. Actually, both Thomas and Chess and we start measuring it *after* 3 months.

Taft: Your ideas about heredity and environment are bound to influence what you say to the parents. Do you say, "Look, here is a basic behavior of the baby, and knowing this will help you understand him a little better"? Or do you say (to yourself), "Maybe the mother's driving him to this kind of behavior, and I have to modify *her*"?

Carey: In the early months, one can say with a fair degree of confidence that this is the way the baby came. As time passes, one becomes less confident. But even at birth, you can't say for sure what's inherited and what's from some intrauterine environmental influence. The principal use of the questionnaires is to give you a better picture of the child's contribution to the parent-child interaction at a given time.

Barnard: The questionnaires show you the child variables that are operating, whether their source is the child's genes, the child's environment, or both.

Brazelton: Aren't you saying essentially that the main uses of the questionnaires are clinical, and that they help you both enter the parent-child relationship and work within it?

Carey: That is the way I use them, yes.

Brazelton: I think the same is true of many tests — even the DDST. They raise the consciousness of parents and clinicians by drawing their attention to things about the child that they otherwise might not see. An assessment is not only a way to identify problems but a way to enter the lives of parent and child and play a role in them.

The Intimate Relationship of Health, Development, and Behavior in the Young Child

by Martin Bax, M.D.

Recurrent "minor" infections and speech delays often occur in the same preschool children, Martin Bax reports, and these children also tend to have behavior problems. Summarizing findings from an experimental health-care program conducted in two London neighborhoods over a 5-year period, Bax emphasizes the need for periodic pediatric examination of all preschool children.

In the discussion following his paper, Bax points out that risk signs have immediate importance as well as possible future significance, and he suggests that pediatricians deal with them on that basis. For example, a 3-year-old who does not talk should be treated for that. The difficulties with reading that may follow years later are almost beside the point.

It has been known for some time that children with a

handicap are more likely than others to have a behavior disorder, presumably because handicapped children are more vulnerable when faced with environmental stress. Most of the studies that demonstrate this fact have been performed with older children who have long-term handicaps. Our clinical experience with hundreds of London children over a 5-year period shows that a close relationship also exists between health problems and developmental and behavior disorders during the preschool years. This finding has implications for the character and timing of health services in the United States as well as in England, despite the different healthcare systems of the two countries.

From 1974 to 1979, we followed the preschool population of two inner-city areas in London. In all, we saw some 870 children and carried out 2,148 examinations. Attendance at our clinics was over 97%. We saw the children for regular examinations at the following ages: 6 weeks, 6 months, 1 year, 1½, 2, 3, and 4½. At each age, we took the child's history and recorded all episodes of illness since the last visit. We also collected data on the child's behavior and development during the period. We then carried out a full pediatric examination of the child, including an observational session.

At all ages, some children were reported as having frequent upper respiratory tract infections (colds, sore throats), frequent lower respiratory tract infections (bronchitis, croup), or frequent otitis media (ear infections). Not surprisingly, there were strong correlations between colds and bronchitis and between colds and ear infections.

We also discovered that children who have frequent infections are much more likely than children who don't to have developmental problems and behavior problems. In addition, children with a developmental problem are likelier than others to have a behavior problem. To illustrate, I will summarize our findings on a very common developmental disorder of the preschool years, speech and language delay.

Table 7. Percentage of Children with
Abnormal Speech and Language

	Possibly abnormal	Definitely abnormal
2 years (N = 296)	17% (50)	5% (14)
3 years (N = 323)	12% (38)	8% (25)
4½ years (N = 269)	7% (19)	5% (13)

Table 8. Percentage of Children
with Common Behavior Problems

	1 year	2 years	3 years	4½ years
Frequent night wakings	27%	21%	21%	16%
Frequent temper tantrums		18%	18%	11%
Frequently very difficult to manage		5%	8%	7%
N =	278	302	331	278

Table 9. Relation Between Speech and Language
Development and Behavior Problems

	Normal	Possibly abnormal	Definitely abnormal
Speech and language at 2 years			
No problem (N = 263)	82% (215)	16% (43)	2% (5)
Behavior problem to parents (N = 33)	55% (18)	21% (7)	24% (8)
			$p = < .001$
Speech and language at 3 years			
No problem (N = 275)	80% (219)	13% (35)	7% (21)
Behavior problem to parents (N = 48)	85% (41)	6% (3)	8% (4)
			Not significant
Speech and language at 4½ years			
No problem (N = 236)	90% (212)	6% (14)	4% (10)
Behavior problem to parents (N = 33)	75% (25)	15% (5)	9% (3)
			$p = < .01$

EAR INFECTIONS AND SPEECH DELAYS. Table 7 gives the percentage of children who showed abnormal speech and language development at ages 2, 3, and 4½. At age 2, we found a highly significant relationship between ear infections in the previous 6 months and definitely delayed speech and language development. At age 3, the percentage of children with ear infections was twice as high in the group with delayed speech as in the normal group, though the findings just failed to reach a statistically significant level.

Table 8 gives the percentage of children with some common behavior problems at ages 1, 2, 3, and 4½. At ages 2, 3, and 4½, there were significant relationships between persistent night waking and ear infections. (Night waking at the time of the infection itself was not included.) In addition, there were highly significant relationships between frequent colds, frequent management difficulties as reported by parents, and frequent temper tantrums.

Table 9 shows the relation between abnormal speech and language and behavior problems at ages 2, 3, and 4½. It is obvious from the table that a disproportionate number of children with speech problems are also presenting behavior problems, especially at ages 2 and 4½.

Children with delayed speech and language development have been shown to do badly in school. The evidence concerning later consequences of behavior disorders is less certain, but there is no doubt that early problems lead to later difficulties in at least some cases.

NEED FOR REGULAR PEDIATRIC EXAMS. Our findings show how closely delayed development is linked to physical illness and strongly support the need for adequate pediatric services for preschool children. The entire population of preschool children in a community should be examined at regular intervals. Our experience has shown us that there is no way to find all the children who need help other than to see and examine them all. Examinations of subpopulations will always miss some important cases. The relatively high rate of behavior disorder at all ages (about 15%) also makes the periodic assessment of all preschool children very worthwhile.

It is extremely difficult to demonstrate the effectiveness of preventive medicine, but we do have data suggesting that children benefit from attending our clinics. First, there are significantly lower rates of speech and language delay in our children than in children seen at 4½ in a control area. Second, children who have been coming to the clinics since early infancy have lower rates of some behavior problems than do children whom we have not been seeing for as long. Such findings, together with parental satisfaction, cause us to believe our service is helpful.

Apart from health-service implications, our experiences have important implications for further research. In this paper I have not examined the relationship between our findings in the children and problems within the families. This topic has considerable interest for our research unit and must be studied if the complex interactions between a child's biological status and environment are to be properly understood.

Taft: How do you explain the correlations between ear infections, speech delay, and behavior problems?

Bax: Chronic ear infections seem often to cause a mild, temporary hearing loss, which leads to a simple delay in speech development — six months to a year. The behavior problems may begin with discomfort caused by the physical illness, or they may stem from the child's frustration over speech difficulties.

Lubchenco: We see a lot of otitis in our tiny prematures, and we also find more speech problems later. We've thought there might be a connection.

Bax: That's quite possible. Small babies are twice as likely as the normal population to have respiratory tract infections. In general, when we look at the backgrounds of children with chronic difficulties, we find low birth weights at about double the rate of small babies in the general population.

Parmelee: Did you talk with mothers about their own lives at all, or only about the children?

Bax: We interviewed the mothers once a year, partly to find out what health facilities and services they wanted offered to them and partly because we were interested in maternal depression. Some studies done 3 or 4 years ago showed that in the United Kingdom mothers with children under age 5 had much higher rates of depression than women the same age who did not have young children. We rated about 20% of the mothers in our sample as moderately or severely depressed. There was a very strong correlation between depression in the mother and temper tantrums or other problem behaviors in the child.

Frankenburg: Home environment correlates with hearing loss, you know, and also with language development and school failure. In our screening study of 10,000 poverty children, we looked not only for hearing problems but for speech problems, eye problems, and developmental problems. We found a lot of speech problems, but we interpreted them as reflecting the poverty circumstances in which the children were growing up. I was surprised at how few children showed hearing losses, but I think now it was because most hearing loss in childhood is transient. At this point I even question the value of screening for hearing loss, since it is almost always temporary. Incidentally, we also found a relationship between the developmental status of the child and whether the child had eye problems. I think the thing to look at is the home environment.

Bax: I agree that home environment is very important, but home environment is a difficult thing for a physician to change.

Frankenburg: That may be. I'm just cautioning you not to assume that there's a cause-effect relationship between hearing loss and speech problems in these children. It may be another factor, like lack of stimulation.

Bax: In the children we saw, ear infections were not class-related. They occurred at about the same rate in all socioeconomic groups. We did find an association between low SES and frequent infections of the lower respiratory tract.

Brazelton: SES keeps cropping up as a major variable, doesn't it? As physicians, we can't change it for people, but we can certainly be conscious of it and work with it as a background variable.

Bax: In our work we found it easier than we had expected to get low SES families to come to the clinic, so that was a pleasant surprise. But you have to be realistic about what you can do to help with class-related problems. For instance, I don't think I can persuade the English government to increase benefits for people out of work.

Brazelton: I was talking about intervention by health-care providers, not by governments.

Parmelee: I would be very disappointed if we didn't think about governments, though. It seems to me that research findings like those we've just heard *should* influence public policy.

Brazelton: Pediatricians and other health-care professionals may be one of the few groups who have a chance to intervene and try to improve outcome for low SES children.

Horowitz: In England they have what amounts to an intervention program on a national scale, through the Health Service. In this country we have only the physician. From the time an infant leaves the hospital till the time the same child appears at school, there is no other high-probability contact with the family except the physician. Even at that, the latest statistics I'm aware of suggest that only half the children in the United States are under medical supervision of any kind.

Frankenburg: I would rather talk about the child's environment than about socioeconomic status, because a health-care professional cannot change socioeconomic status but can change some environmental variables.

Lubchenco: Some factors in SES have nothing to do with money.

Frankenburg: As we all know, families with high incomes can have very deprived children, and poverty circumstances don't necessarily mean you're depriving your child.

Denhoff: Still, a lack of money does keep a lot of people from getting good health care. There are quite a few health-care programs for low-income families set up at the community level. But most of these programs are disease-oriented, whereas we're talking about preventive medicine.

Bax: The way I see it, a 3-year-old who doesn't talk has something wrong with him, and something should be done for that child now. I know that 40% of 3-year-olds who do not talk are going to have reading difficulties later, but I would treat the 3-year-old for nontalking and wait a few years to worry about the reading. Sometimes I think I don't really believe in risk and prediction. I believe in treating abnormalities in children when I find them at the time I find them.

A Sensory-Motor Enrichment Program

by Eric Denhoff, M.D.

An unusual feature of the Meeting Street School program for infants with developmental impairments or delays is that treatment is aimed at enhancing existing sensory-motor strengths rather than at alleviating deficits. Sensory-motor enrichment for the child is only part of the program, however. Denhoff gives equal importance to supporting the parents, both through training and emotionally.

Intervention programs almost always have positive effects for parents, and through them for the child. No one at our conference disputed this claim, and many explicitly endorsed it. As the socioemotional benefits of intervention become more widely recognized and appreciated, Denhoff suggests, the present low rate of physician referrals can be expected to rise.

In the traditional approach to the treatment of infants with neuromotor problems, an initial sensory-motor assessment is followed by physical, occupational, and speech therapies to reduce impairment in problem areas. At the Meeting Street School in Providence, Rhode Island, we use a different approach. Repeated comprehensive assessments are coupled with treatment aimed at reinforcing sensory and neuromotor strengths.

A newborn infant's tactile-kinesthetic awareness and capacity for visual scanning often are intact unless the child has suffered intense and prolonged oxygen deprivation. If the caretaker knows how to interpret the baby's signals, these sensory pathways can be used to permit meaningful contact with the environment. Clinical evidence shows that recovery can be fostered by means of these primitive routes.

An example is provided by two spastic hemiplegic youngsters, brother and sister. We have observed over the years that the atypical gait associated with spastic hemiplegia can be modified by physical therapy, bracing, or orthopedic surgery. Seizures can be controlled by anticonvulsant medication, strabismus by glasses or surgical correction, and attentional deficit by behavior modification or psychostimulant medication. But a persistent barrier to academic and life adjustment remains: a flexed wrist and ineffective hand usage, often compounded by loss of tactile-kinesthetic awareness in the affected hand.

I invited the parents of these impaired babies to participate in a home enrichment program that emphasized improving sensory input. At the start, I asked the parents always to present material to the child's left hand for touching and feeling, and then to encourage motor action with the impaired right hand. These instructions were based on Wittleson's notion that the right hemisphere of the brain (left hand) is better designed to take in sensory information, and the left hemisphere (right hand) is designed to act upon such information. I encouraged bilateral hand use and insisted on use of the impaired hand in all activities.

From these children I learned that much of the crying and fussing seen in neurologically impaired infants comes from frustration at not being able to complete tasks successfully. Our enrichment program was designed to help the parents help the infants derive satisfaction by improving their performance.

Guidance for the parents was another important part of the program. I discussed with them the probable difficulties the children would have with self-image, peers, and school. Although our critics believed we were creating problems rather than preventing them, as the children grew older they did encounter many of the complications we had anticipated and discussed with their parents.

Both children, but especially the boy, seemed to compensate readily for the deficient hand. He did not develop impaired sensory function and could manage the use of items ranging from a basketball to a ball-point pen. His sister, though more involved anatomically according to CAT scan, had more difficulty establishing a good self-image than achieving good penmanship. With strong family support and teacher understanding, she has gained self-confidence and rebounded into the mainstream of life activities.

Infant enrichment programs aid not only babies but parents, because they provide positive direction and support while attenuating grief-anger reactions. The Committee on Children with Handicaps of the American Academy of Pediatrics supports enrichment programs because they provide a tangible family support system as well as an opportunity for the pediatrician to arrive at a realistic appraisal of infant status and family capability.

THE MEETING STREET SCHOOL PROGRAM. During the past 20 years, more than 2,000 infants have been enrolled in the Meeting Street School Parent Program for Developmental Management. The program teaches parents a series of sensory, perceptual, motor, language, and social interventions to use with developmentally jeopardized infants in an effort to help them interact with the environment more effectively. The parents provide the enrichments under the supervision of a trained interventionist, who in turn is supported by a developmental team. The guidelines followed by interventionists are shown in Table 10, and the management program for early infancy is summarized in Table 11.

Table 10. Guidelines for Interventionists

1. Do not interfere with the natural timetable of skill emergence.
2. Initiate enrichments at the baby's level and on the baby's terms.
3. The order of interventions is: social-emotional, communication, perceptual-motor, motor.
4. Sensory awareness precedes motor output.
5. Parent grief reactions are often camouflaged. Understand, help, reassure, but be honest and realistic.

Table 11. Enrichment Program for Early Infancy

Interactions	Early needs	Instruments
Mother-infant	Rocking, cuddling, touching, fondling, rubbing, talking to	Rocking chair, toweling, self
Father-infant	Motion through handling, in varied body positions	Hassock or barrel, self
Sensory	Visual, tactile, auditory, smell, taste, eye-hand	"Comfort me mitt," mobiles, lights, sounds, textures
Feeding-language	Sucking, chewing, swallowing, tasting, smelling, sounding	Primitive reflexes, reinforcement with nipples, foods

The interventionist encourages the parents to provide enrichments in a structured manner in order to hold the child's attention and avoid habituation (a decline in responsiveness). Animal studies suggest that sensory stimulation causes receptor neurons to expand in size or increase in number, but if habituation occurs there may be a slowing of neuronal development. While controversial, these studies imply that a lack of interest can have a direct influence on brain growth in the very young animal.

A successful program depends on a proper match between parents and interventionist based on therapeutic expertise, perceptiveness, gentleness, and responsiveness to needs. Mutual caring is important, and the interventionist must develop a trust relationship with the family.

The Meeting Street School is one of six early intervention programs in Rhode Island, serving about one-fourth of the infants enrolled in such programs. In 1978, 51 infants were referred to us: 22 for developmental disabilities (cerebral palsy, hypotonia, Down's syndrome, hydrocephalus, and visual impairment), 28 for developmental delay, and 1 for behavior disorder.

NEW CHALLENGES. The emergence of intensive perinatal care as an integral part of pediatrics has significantly increased the salvageability rate for very high-risk babies. Most high-risk, low birth-weight infants show transient abnormal central nervous system signs between 4 and 12 months, which then resolve so that the infants appear to be growing up normally. Only 10 to 20% of infants weighing less than 2500 grams at birth develop obvious neurological problems, assuming they receive sophisticated care.

Consequently, pediatricians are inclined to adopt a wait-and-see attitude instead of making early referrals to intervention and enrichment programs. In Rhode Island in 1978, the mean age of infants at the time of referral was 13.8 months. This is disconcerting, because it postpones treatment until an age when adverse behavior patterns may already be established.

Community health programs and social workers refer the most cases; private pediatricians, the fewest. At the Women and Infants Hospital in Rhode Island, where the intensive care unit population averages 1,000 cases a year, only 50 infants a year are referred to enrichment programs because of suspicious neurological findings. In Rhode Island in 1978, less than 30% of infants with low birth weights were enrolled in intervention programs, and only 1% of all live births regardless of weight.

Among the high-risk infants who tend never to reach enrichment programs are the babies of unmarried teenage mothers. Many of these babies are emotionally passive and are candidates for neglect, deprivation, and abuse. Very young mothers are involved in about one-third of the cases of child abuse in Rhode Island. Infants of teenage mothers would benefit greatly from sensory enrichments, and their mothers from the support that our program and others like it offer.

Partly because disabilities are individualized, controlled outcome studies showing that enrichment "works" are not feasible. However, the clinical evidence is indisputable that such programs help reinforce tottering relationships between infants with suspected developmental problems and their worried parents. When progress exceeds expectations, as often happens with stimulation, everyone reacts with pride. This can be the start of a lifelong trust-based relationship between child and family, and the beginning of the development of independence.

Barnard: I'm surprised at the low referral rate in your state, with such a fine program and good reputation. What's behind it, do you think?

Denhoff: Some physicians resist referring infants to intervention programs because they think the programs make unrealistic promises about the child's progress instead of viewing them as a system of family support.

Barnard: Your description clearly shows that you give

high priority to supporting the parents. This is in line with my own feeling that the family is the basic health-care unit and that, really, our job is to support them.

Brazelton: Some physicians are slow to refer for a kind of competitive reason — they are reluctant to give up providing that support themselves. This feeling is based on real caring about the people they're working with.

Denhoff: Another reason is the lack of good outcome studies. We can't show for sure that intervention programs do more to facilitate recovery than good mothering. This is what physicians often ask: How do you know that what you're doing is better than just good mothering? Well, we don't know. But judging by the criterion of parental acceptance, our program has a success rate of about 90%. Most of our parents say they couldn't do without it.

Taft: In considering whether intervention is beneficial or not, I think we should recognize that we are discussing two different populations. One is the high-risk infant, the infant who may develop a problem later on. The other is the damaged child whose problem has already been diagnosed. I think there is more acceptance in the professional community of the value of intervention for the latter group.

Denhoff: The only cases I see that don't make progress with intervention are the severely deprived, resuscitated hypoxic infants, the very tiny ones who weren't expected to survive at all. With the others, progress does occur. It may not occur exactly as we wish, but the children do grow. Their social and emotional growth is especially impressive.

Brazelton: It has been brought out repeatedly at this conference that we can do more to help children with damaged nervous systems recover socially and emotionally than neurologically or motorically. I've felt strongly all the way through that we were talking about separating neurological recovery from socio-emotional recovery as a goal, because they have very different connotations both from a developmental standpoint and from a research standpoint.

Als: Somehow there's the notion that only motor output matters. We need to see social and emotional behavior as an equally important part of the integrated capacity of the nervous system.

Duffy: Yes — and the brain is involved in "psychosocial" behavior as well as in movement, of course. For example, a young child who was brought to me recently for irritability turned out to have a subtle right-hemisphere lesion. In older children and adults, the right hemisphere is known to be the part of the brain that perceives context, emotion, Gestalt. I talked with the mother, and it was perfectly clear that this child could not pick up on other people's contextual cues — tone of voice, facial expression, and the like. For instance, he had a lot of trouble telling when his mother was getting angry with him, so he often misbehaved. Children with similar lesions in the left hemisphere have the opposite problem: They pick up on emotional cues very well, so they seem to understand what the parent is telling them, but in fact they don't understand detailed verbal statements at all.

Parmelee: How old are these children?

Duffy: I've seen the right-hemisphere lesion from the teen years all the way down to 2 or 3. Strategies that suggest hemispheric damage may also be present in infants under a year, but that's only a suspicion of mine — I'm not certain.

Brazelton: Well, I feel very positive about health-care professionals' attitude toward intervention programs. The Academy of Pediatrics has just established its first new committee in 5 years, and it's called the Committee on Psychosocial Development of Children and Families. I think this reflects a need that is beginning to identify itself on many different levels.

Horowitz: If you look at the outcome literature, you don't find studies proving that procedure X leads to improvement Y, but at least there are no programs that have been shown to hurt children. Sometimes you find no difference, and sometimes you find improvement.

Bax: Still, I think one should be very cautious about interfering in people's child-rearing unless one has really reliable evidence that one is helping.

McCall: I'm not so sure. Perhaps the research scientist can afford to say, "Well, I'll wait 10 years until the data are in," but there are other folks out there who want the best advice and assistance that they can get *now*.

Brazelton: I agree, Bob, that we really can't wait for incontrovertible evidence, and that research on outcomes has to follow at this point.

Parmelee: The scientists and others who control government funding seem to say we have to study the outcome measures first. The ones we've been using — particularly the Stanford-Binet — haven't been adequate, so now the issue is what outcome measure we want to look at. For example, we've talked a great deal today about how much intervention programs help families. We have to be able to show that, and we also have to be able to show that helping the family helped the child.

Barnard: It's such a value-laden area, though. I remember a study showing that a certain project led to much less marital disruption in the families involved, and some people criticized it by saying, "Well, what's so good about families staying together?"

Brazelton: The reality is that well-controlled outcome studies are very difficult to conduct. I'm not sure any of us could run one that had the controls we would like. But we do have a wealth of clinical evidence favoring intervention.

Denhoff: I agree, and I think the others around this table would, too. But we've heard many viewpoints expressed here, Berry. Before we close, let me ask if you would summarize the areas of agreement that stand out in your mind.

Brazelton: All of us seem to believe that the at-risk infant demonstrates an impressive and amazing amount of recuperability, particularly under optimal environmental conditions. All of us feel that early intervention by professionals can help caring, but disturbed, parents provide a more favorable environment.

The opportunity to intervene early, before a failure pattern of pathology is established, must certainly be a clinician's goal. The dangers of labeling or of overidentification of disordered children are not great when an intervention is appropriate to the parents and to the child — though deciding on the precise ingredients of such intervention would require another conference.

The confusion between prediction and individual cases has dogged this round table. Accurate prediction is not the main purpose of assessment if our goal is early intervention and support for the families of disordered infants. For assessment and identification are of no value unless they enhance our capacity to assist in correcting the situation — thereby invalidating predictions based on our assessments. The goal of an assessment should be appropriate intervention, not correct prediction. I would hope we could aim for a future conference in which we establish the mutable aspects of high-risk children and families, and further explore the role that professionals might play in enhancing positive change.

References and Suggested Readings

Als, H., and Brazelton, T.B. A new model of assessing the behavioral organization in preterm and fullterm infants: two case studies. *Journal of the American Academy of Child Psychiatry* 20:239-63. 1981.

Als, H., Lester, B.M., and Brazelton, T.B. Dynamics of the behavioral organization of the premature infant: a theoretical perspective. In *Infants born at risk: behavior and development,* eds. T.M. Field, A.M. Sostek, S. Goldberg, and H.H. Shuman. Jamaica, N.Y.: Spectrum. 1979.

Als, H., Lester, B.M., Tronick, E., and Brazelton, T.B. Towards a research instrument for the assessment of preterm infants' behavior. In *Theory and research in behavioral pediatrics,* Vol. 1, eds. H.E. Fitzgerald, B.M. Lester, and M.W. Yogman. New York: Plenum. In press.

Anderson, J.E. The limitations of infant and preschool tests in the measurement of intelligence. *Journal of Psychology* 8:351-79. 1939.

Bax, M., and Hart, H. Health needs of pre-school children. *Archives of Diseases of Childhood* 51:848-52. 1976.

Bax, M., Hart, H., and Jenkins, S. Assessment of speech and language development in the young child. *Pediatrics* 66, No. 3.

Bayley, N. Mental growth during the first three years: a developmental study of 61 children by repeated tests. *Genetic Psychology Monographs* 14:1-92. 1933.

Bayley, N. Some increasing parent-child similarities during the growth of children. *Journal of Educational Psychology* 45:1-21. 1954.

Birns, B., and Golden, M. Prediction of intellectual performance at three years from infant tests and personality measures. *Merrill-Palmer Quarterly* 18:53-58. 1972.

Brazelton, T.B. Assessment techniques for enhancing infant development. Presented at the Clinical Infant Programs, Washington, D.C. 1979.

Brazelton, T.B. Neonatal Behavioral Assessment Scale. National Spastics Monographs No. 50. Philadelphia: Lippincott. 1973.

Broman, S. H. Perinatal anoxia and cognitive development in early childhood. In *Infants born at risk: behavior and development,* eds. T.M. Field, A.M. Sostek, S. Goldberg, and H.H. Shuman, Jamaica, N.Y.: Spectrum. 1979.

Carey, W.B. Clinical appraisal of temperament. In *Developmental disabilities: theory, assessment, and intervention,* eds. M. Lewis and L. Taft. Jamaica, N.Y.: SP Medical and Scientific Books. 1981.

Carey, W.B. The importance of temperament-environment interaction for child health and development. In *The uncommon child,* eds. M. Lewis and L. Rosenblum. New York: Plenum. 1981.

Carey, W.B., and McDevitt, S.C. Revision of the Infant Temperament Questionnaire. *Pediatrics* 61:735-39. 1978.

Carr, J. *Young children with Down's syndrome: their development, upbringing, and effect on their families.* London: Butterworths. 1975.

Cattell, P. *The measurement of intelligence in infants and young children.* New York: Science Press. 1940. Reprinted by the Psychological Corp., 1960.

Cavanaugh, M.C., Cohen, I., Dunphy, D., Ringwell, E.A., and Goldberg, I.D. Prediction from the Cattell Infant Intelligence Scale. *Journal of Consulting Psychology* 21:33-37. 1957.

Denhoff E. Assessment of at-risk infant and early stimulation. In *The at-risk infant,* ed. S. Harel. Princeton: Excerpta Medica. 1980.

Denhoff, E. Current status of infant stimulation or enrichment programs for children with developmental disabilities. *Pediatrics* 67:32-37. 1981.

Denhoff, E. The natural life history of children with M.B.D. In *Minimal brain dysfunction,* eds. F. de la Cruz, B.H. Fox, and R.H. Roberts. New York: Academy of Sciences. 1973.

Denhoff, E., and Hyman, I. Meeting Street School Project parent programs for developmental management. In *Intervention strategies for high risk infants and children,* ed. T.D. Tjossem. Baltimore: Univ. Park Press. 1976.

Dicks-Mireaux, M.J. Development of intelligence of children with Down's syndrome. *American Journal of Mental Deficiency* 63:307-11. 1958.

Drillien, C.M. Longitudinal study of growth and development of prematurely and maturely born children: VII. Mental development 2-5 years. *Archives of Diseases of Childhood* 36:233-40. 1961.

Drillien, C.M., Thomson, A.J.M., and Bargoyne, K. Low birthweight children at early school-age: a longitudinal study. *Developmental Medicine and Child Neurology* 22:26-47. 1980.

Dubowitz, L.M.S., Dubowitz, V., and Goldberg, C. Clinical assessment of gestational age in the newborn infant. *Journal of Pediatrics* 77:1. 1970.

Duffy, F.H., Burchfiel, J.L., and Lombroso, C.T. Brain electrical activity mapping (BEAM): a method for extending the clinical utility of EEG and evoked potential data. *Annals of Neurology* 5:309-21.

Duffy, F.H., Denckla, M.B., Bartels, P.H., and Sandini, G. Dyslexia: regional differences in brain electrical activity by topographic mapping. *Annals of Neurology* 7:412-20. 1980.

Duffy, F.H., Denckla, M.B., Bartels, P.H., Sandini, G., and Kiessling, L.S. Dyslexia: automated diagnosis by computerized classification of brain electrical activity. *Annals of Neurology* 7:421-28. 1980.

Elardo, R., Bradley, R., and Caldwell, B.M. The relation of infants' home environments to mental test performance from six to thirty-six months: a longitudinal analysis. *Child Development* 46:71-76. 1975.

Erickson, M.T. The predictive validity of the Cattell Intelligence Scale for young mentally retarded children. *American Journal of Mental Deficiency* 72: 728-33. 1968.

Escalona, S.K., and Moriarty, A. Prediction of school-age intelligence from infant tests. *Child Development* 32:597-605. 1961.

Fillmore, E.A. Iowa tests for young children. *Univ. of Iowa Studies in Child Welfare* 11:1-58. 1936.

Fishler, K., Graleker, B.V., and Koch, R. The predictability of intelligence with Gesell Developmental Scales in mentally retarded infants and young children. *American Journal of Mental Deficiency* 69: 515-25. 1964-65.

Fishman, M., and Palkes, H. The validity of psychometric testing in children with congenital malformations of the central nervous system. *Developmental Medicine and Child Neurology* 16:180-85. 1974.

Fitzhardinge, E., Kalman, E., Ashby, S., and Pope, K.I. Present status of the infant of very low birth weight treated in a referral neonatal intensive care unit in 1974. *Major mental handicap: methods and costs of prevention.* North Holland: Elsevier. 1978.

Frankenburg, W.K., and Camp, B.W. *Pediatric screening tests.* Springfield, Ill.: Charles C. Thomas. 1975.

Frankenburg, W.K., Coons, C.E., and Ker, C. Screening infants and preschoolers to identify school learning problems (DDST and HOME scale). Alice Hayden's Symposium Proceedings. Baltimore: Univ. Park Press.

Gesell, A., and Ilg, F. L. *Infant and child in the culture of today.* New York: Harper. 1943.

Goffeney, B., Henderson, N.B., and Butler, B.V. Negro-white, male-female eight-month and developmental scores compared with seven-year WISC and Bender test scores. *Child Development* 42:595-604. 1971.

Goodman, J., and Cameron, J. The meaning of IQ constancy in young retarded children. *Journal of Genetic Psychology* 132:109-11. 1978.

Hart, H., Bax, M., and Jenkins, S. The use of the child health clinic. *Archives of Diseases of Childhood.* In press.

Hindley, C.B. Stability and change in abilities up to five years: group trends. *Journal of Child Psychology and Psychiatry* 6:85-99. 1965.

Honzik, M.P., Macfarlane, J.W., and Allen, L. The stability of mental test performance between two and eighteen years. *Journal of Experimental Education* 18:309-24. 1948.

Horowitz, F.D. Normal and abnormal child development. In *Early intervention — a team approach,* eds. K.E. Allen, V.A. Holm, and R.L. Schiefelbusch. Baltimore: Univ. Park Press. 1978.

Horowitz, F.D. Intervention and its effects on early development: what model of development is appropriate? In *Life-span developmental psychology: intervention,* eds. R.R. Turner and H.W. Reese. New York: Academic Press. 1980.

Horowitz, F.D. Toward a functional analysis of individual differences. Presidential address to the Division of Developmental Psychology, American Psychological Assn. meeting, Toronto, 1978.

Hubel, D.H., and Wiesel, T.N. The period of susceptibility to the physiological effects of unilateral eye closure in kittens. *Journal of Physiology* 206:419-36. 1970.

Hubel, D.H., and Wiesel, T.N. Receptive fields, binocular interaction and functional architecture in the cat's visual cortex. *Journal of Physiology* 160:106-54. 1962.

Hunt, J.V. Longitudinal research: a method for studying the intellectual development of high-risk preterm infants. In *Infants born at risk: behavior and development,* eds. T.M. Field, M.M. Sostek, S. Goldberg, and H.H. Shuman. Jamaica, N.Y.: Spectrum. 1979.

Ireton, H., Thwing, E., and Gravem, H. Infant mental development and neurological status, family socio-economic status, and intelligence at age four. *Child Development* 41:937-46. 1970.

Kangas, J., Butler, B.V., and Goffeney, B. Relationship between preschool intelligence, maternal intelligence, and infant behavior. Second Scientific Session, Collaborative Study on Cerebral Palsy, Mental Retardation, and Other Neurological and Sensory Disorders of Infancy and Childhood. U.S. Dept. of Health, Education, and Welfare, Public Health Service, Pt. 2, 91-102. 1966.

Klackenberg-Larsson, I., and Stensson, J. Data on the mental development during the first five years. In The development of children in a Swedish urban community: a prospective longitudinal study. *Acta Paediatrica Scandinavica,* Supplement 187, IV, Almqvist and Wiksell, Stockholm. 1968.

Knobloch, H., and Pasamanick, B. An evaluation of the consistency and predictive value of the 40 week Gesell development schedule. In *Child development and child psychiatry,* eds. C. Shagass and B. Pasamanick. Washington, D.C.: American Psychiatric Assn. 1960.

Kopp, C.B., and McCall, R.B. Stability and instability in mental performance among normal, at-risk, and handicapped infants and children. In *Life-span de-*

velopment and behavior, Vol. 4, eds. P.B. Baltes and O.C. Brim, Jr., New York: Academic Press. In press.

Lashley, K.S. Factors limiting recovery after central nervous system lesions. *Journal of Nervous and Mental Disorders* 88: 733-55. 1938.

Lester, B.M. Behavioral assessment of the infant. In *Follow-up of the high risk newborn: a practical approach,* ed. E. Sell. Springfield, Ill.: Charles C. Thomas. 1980.

Lester, B.M. The continuity of change in infant development. Presented at the Bienniel Meeting of the Society for Research in Child Development, Boston, 1981.

Lester, B.M., Emory, E., Hoffman, S., and Eitzman, D. A multivariate study on the effects of high risk factors on performance on the Brazelton Neonatal Assessment Scale. *Child Development* 47:237-41. 1976.

Lewis, M., and Rosenblum, L. *The uncommon child.* New York: Plenum. 1981.

Lewis, M., and Taft, L., eds. *Developmental disabilities: theory, assessment, and intervention.* Jamaica, N.Y.: SP Medical and Scientific Books. 1981.

Linn, P.L. Newborn environments and mother-infant interactions. Dissertation, Univ. of Kansas. 1979.

Lubchenco, L.O. *The high risk infant.* Philadelphia: Saunders. 1976.

Luria, A.R. *Traumatic aphasia.* The Hague: Mouton. 1970.

McCall, R.B., Hogarty, P.S., and Hurlburt, N. Transitions in infant sensorimotor development and the prediction of childhood IQ. *American Psychologist* 27:728-48. 1972.

McCall, R.B. The development of intellectual functioning in infancy and the prediction of later IQ. In

Handbook of infant development, ed. J. D. Osofsky. New York: Wiley. 1979.

McCall, R.B. Toward an epigenetic conception of mental development in the first three years of life. In *Origins of intelligence,* ed. M. Lewis. New York: Plenum. 1976.

McDevitt, S.C., and Carey, W.B. The measurement of temperament in 3-7 year old children. *Journal of Child Psychology and Psychiatry* 19:245-53. 1978.

Meyer, P.M. Recovery of function following lesions of the subcortex and neocortex. In *Plasticity and recovery of function in the central nervous system,* eds. D.G. Stein, J.J. Rosen, and N. Butters. New York: Academic Press. 1974.

Moore, R.Y. Central regeneration and recovery of function: the problem of collateral reinervation. In *Plasticity and recovery of function in the central nervous system,* eds. D.G. Stein, J.J. Rosen, and N. Butters. New York: Academic Press. 1974.

Moore, T. Language and intelligence: a longitudinal study of the first eight years. Part I. Patterns of development in boys and girls. *Human Development* 10:88-106. 1967.

Nelson, C., and Horowitz, F.D. The short-term behavioral sequelae of neonatal jaundice (hyperbilirubinemia) and phototherapy. In press.

Nelson, K.B., and Broman, S.H. Perinatal risk factors in children with serious motor and mental handicaps. *Annals of Neurology* 2:371-77. 1977.

Nelson, V.L., and Richards, T.W. Studies in mental development: III. Performance of twelve-month-old children on the Gesell schedule and its predictive value for mental status at two and three years. *Journal of Genetic Psychology* 54:181-91. 1939.

Parmelee, A.H. Planning intervention for infants at high risk identified by developmental evaluation. In

Research to practice in mental retardation, Vol. 1, *Care and Intervention,* ed. P. Mittler. Baltimore: Univ. Park Press. 1977.

Parmelee, A.H., Beckwith, L., Cohen, S.E., Sigman, M. Social influences on infants at medical risk for behavioral difficulties. In *Proceedings of the First World Congress on Infant Psychiatry,* eds. J. Call and E. Gallenson. New York: Basic Books. 1981.

Prechtl, H.F.R. Assessment methods for the newborn infant: a critical evaluation. In *Psychobiology of the human newborn,* ed. P. Stratton. New York: Wiley. In press.

Prechtl, H.F.R. The neurological examination of the full-term newborn infant, 2nd revised and enlarged version. *Clinics in Developmental Medicine,* no. 63. London: Heinemann. 1977.

Prechtl, H.F.R. The optimality concept. Editorial. *Early Human Development* 4:201-05.

Saint-Anne Dargassies, S. *The development of the nervous system in the foetus.* Vevey, Switzerland: Documents scientifiques Guigoz. 1968.

Saint-Anne Dargassies, S. The normal and abnormal neurological examination of the neonate: silent neurological abnormalities. In *Advances in perinatal neurology,* Vol. I, eds. R. Korobkin and C. Guilleminault. Jamaica, N.Y.: SP Medical and Scientific Books. 1979.

Saint-Anne Dargassies, S. *Neurological development in the full term and premature neonate.* New York: Excerpta Medica. 1977.

Saint-Anne Dargassies, S. Neurological maturation of the premature infant of 28 to 41 weeks gestational age. In *Human development,* ed. F. Falkner, pp. 305-26. Philadelphia: Saunders. 1966.

Saint James-Roberts, I. Neurological plasticity, recovery from brain insult and child development. In *Advances in child development.* New York: Academic Press. 1979.

Sameroff, A.J., and Chandler, M.J. Reproductive risk and the continuum of caretaking casualty. In *Review of child development research,* Vol. 4, ed. F.D. Horowitz. Chicago: Univ. of Chicago Press. 1975.

Sander, L. W. Issues in early mother-child interaction. *Journal of the American Academy of Child Psychiatry* 1:141-66. 1962.

Share, J., Webb, A., and Koch, R. A preliminary investigation of the early development status of mongoloid infants. *American Journal of Mental Deficiency* 66:238-41. 1961-62.

Siegel, L., Saigal, S., Rosenbaum, P., Young, A., Berenbaum, S., and Stoskopt, B. Correlates and predictors of cognitive and language development of very low birth weight infants. Dept. of Psychiatry and Pediatrics, McMaster Univ. Medical Centre. 1979.

Sigman, M., and Parmelee, A.H. Longitudinal evaluation of the high-risk infant. In *Infants born at risk: behavior and development,* eds. T.M. Field, A.M. Sostek, S. Goldberg, and H.H. Shuman. Jamaica, N.Y.: Spectrum. 1979.

Thomas, A., and Chess, S. *Temperament and development.* New York: Brunner-Mazel. 1977.

Thomas, A., Chess, S., and Birch, H.G. *Behavioral individuality in early childhood.* New York: New York Univ. Press. 1963.

van Doorninck, W.J., Dick, N.P., Frankenburg, W.K., Liddell, T.N., and Lampe, J.M. Infant and preschool developmental screening and later school performance. Paper presented at the Society for Pediatric Research, St. Louis. 1976.

Werner, E.E., Honzik, M.P., and Smith, R.S. Prediction of intelligence and achievement at ten years from 20 months pediatric and psychologic examinations. *Child Development* 39:1063-75. 1968.